Hearing
Better

*Understanding Your Hearing And
Ear Care Options*

by

John M. Burkey, M.A., CCC/A
William H. Lippy, M.D.
Arnold G. Schuring, M.D.
Franklin M. Rizer, M.D.

Universal Publishers/uPUBLISH.com
Parkland, Florida

For those who find themselves
disadvantaged in a hearing world.

Hearing Better:
Understanding Your Hearing And Ear Care Options

John M. Burkey, William H. Lippy,
Arnold G. Schuring, Franklin M. Rizer

published by
Universal Publishers/uPUBLISH.com
Parkland, Florida
USA • 1999

ISBN: 1-58112-823-1

www.upublish.com/books/burkey.htm

**Library of Congress
Cataloging-in-Publication Data**

Hearing better : understanding your hearing
and ear care options / by John M. Burkey
. . . [et al.].
p. 161   cm.
ISBN 1-58112-823-1
1. Hearing disorders Popular Work.
2. Hearing aids. 3. Deaf-
-Rehabilitation. I. Burkey, John M.,
1959-   .
RF300.H433   1999
617.8—dc21   99-37809
                                      CIP

Contents

Foreword

Through 99.9% of recorded history there were no safe or effective treatments for hearing loss. People who were born deaf stayed deaf. Those who developed hearing loss, did not get better. Infection in the ear did not only affect hearing, but was, at times, life threatening or fatal. The development of antibiotics began to change this. Ear infections could be treated or cured and associated hearing losses reduced or eliminated. The operative microscope came into use supplying illumination and magnification and allowed the surgeon to work with both hands. So, surgery for ear problems became a viable option due to the operating microscope and antibiotics. The operating microscope made delicate surgery on the small structures of the ear practical, while antibiotics lowered the risk of postoperative infection and complications.

Thirty-seven years ago, I began practicing medicine. It was an exciting time. Microscopic surgery was brand new, and it offered great promise for repairing the ravages of disease including some that cause hearing loss. One of these new surgical treatments (stapedectomy) was to become my specialty. In the years since, this procedure improved or restored hearing to millions of people worldwide who had the ear disease otosclerosis. Prior to the development of this procedure, these people would have been condemned to a life of hearing loss.

During my years of practice, numerous medical and surgical procedures have been developed for the treatment of hearing loss. Some hearing losses can be completely corrected. Others can be greatly reduced so they present less of a handicap. There are additionally people whose hearing loss cannot be corrected, but medical treatment is needed to minimize or prevent further loss. Unfortunately, not all hearing losses can be treated or corrected medically, but with

4

every year, more and more can. Today, even the totally deaf are not without help. They can have hearing restored through the surgical implantation of a device called a cochlear implant.

When people think about hearing loss, the first thing many think of is hearing aids. They are often unaware that there are medical and surgical treatments that can sometimes eliminate the need for hearing aids altogether. Continued improvements in hearing aids are making them more useful and comfortable than ever before. However, instead of hearing aids, people should first think about whether a hearing loss can be fixed or whether steps need to be taken to prevent their hearing from becoming worse.

I am thrilled to have had the opportunity to contribute to this book. This remains an exciting time for those of us involved in the treatment of hearing loss and ear problems. More can be done today than ever before. Very few of the hearing impaired cannot be helped to hear better with medical treatments, surgical procedures or through the use of hearing aids. *Hearing Better: Understanding Your Hearing And Ear Care Options* presents a balanced overview of the problems associated with hearing loss and the wide range of treatments available. It is informative and easy to read. It should be a valuable guide for those interested in preserving or improving their ability to hear.

William H. Lippy, M.D.

Introduction

Few quality of life and health concerns have received as little public attention as hearing. With the possible exception of a hearing screening in elementary or preschool, the entire concept of hearing and hearing loss is largely ignored in private and public schools. The situation is little better for those who had the opportunity for a university education. Students can count themselves among the more fortunate if they learned the basic structure and function of the ear in an anatomy or health class. The majority only learn the part they need for trivia games (the three smallest bones in the human body are located in the middle ear). We are not taught what we should hear, what might interfere with the things we are trying to hear, what is likely to damage our hearing, or a great number of other hearing related facts that might actually be of practical use. We certainly are not given a clue as to whom to contact if we suspect a hearing problem.

For the majority of us, our hearing related education comes courtesy of television, radio, magazines and newspapers. More specifically, the bulk of this information comes to us through the advertisements in these sources. Rather than the people most knowledgeable or best educated explaining what could or would be helpful for us to know, it is often the people with the largest marketing budget presenting what they want us to buy. The purpose of this book was to provide an alternate source for hearing related information. We wished to share our education and clinical experience with a wider audience than available in our practice alone.

Hearing Better: Understanding Your Hearing And Ear Care Options discusses the basics about ears and hearing as well as new medical and technological advances. It also includes a number of hearing related topics that we feel are important, that are likely to be considered interesting, or are commonly misunderstood. Each topic is discussed in a manner and style similar to what might be said to a patient in our office. Topics are briefly explained, as well as why they are important and how they might affect an individual. Regardless of the topic, terminology is kept to a minimum.

Anyone planning to see an ear specialist for the first time should benefit from the information provided in the following pages. The different ear professionals are introduced, their qualifications and the services they render explained. Also provided is the background information necessary to help understand what these professionals may find. By being informed, it is possible for a person to become more of an active participant in the decision-making about their own health.

Those who have previously undergone a complete ear and hearing evaluation will also benefit from the information provided. In the era of HMOs and managed care, physicians and other health care professionals rarely have time to discuss all of the problems associated with hearing loss. This book fills in some of the gaps. Additionally, new advances in the treatment of hearing loss are constantly taking place. Some of the procedures and treatments discussed were not available just a few years ago. This new information lets people catch up on what is currently available.

Even people who are not experiencing any hearing difficulties, but are concerned about their hearing heath can benefit from this book. They can discover the greatest dangers to their hearing and how to avoid them. They can also discover ways to make better use of their hearing, to augment it, or reach beyond what nature provided.

Hearing Better was arranged for easy reading. Some of the topics include the basics of hearing, common concerns, ear and hearing professionals and current methods of hearing care. These topics are intended to be read as a whole. Since the ability to hear is so delicately interwoven with so many

7

aspects of a person's life, it is important to understand an individual's hearing within a wide context. Reading the book as a whole provides this context. However, it is possible to skip over information on particular ear diseases or age groups that may not be of interest. A glossary of terms that might be encountered during a visit to an ear professional is included for reference.

Chapter One: The Basics

Anatomy Of The Ear (Abridged Version)

In order to talk about the ear, it is probably necessary to describe some of the parts and explain what they do. However, even for people interested in the ear, this can be less than exciting reading. The ear has many parts. They are given descriptive names from archaic languages leaving people with a collective response of "What?". Fortunately, it is not necessary to memorize every part or landmark of the ear. This would be of little value for the majority. Additionally, describing every nook and cranny of the ear using the appropriate terminology could quite possibly weaken or take away the will to read further. We do not wish to do that here. We will therefore present the abridged version.

For anatomic purposes, the ear is divided into three parts. The outer ear is the first part. This includes the portion of the ear you can see and the ear canal. The middle ear is the second part. It includes the eardrum, ear bones and the cavity surrounding these structures. The third part of the ear is called the inner ear and contains the organs for both hearing and balance. There is also a nerve that carries sound from the inner ear to the brain, but it is not usually considered part of the ear.

The outer part of the ear needs little description. It may vary slightly in size, shape or color, but generally looks about the same from person to person. Despite someone having gone to the trouble to name the many curves, bumps and other landmarks of the outer ear, they serve little function with the possible exception of the earlobes. Women use these as a convenient place to store their jewelry (some men too). The ear canal which is additionally considered part of the outer ear also needs little description. This is the part of the ear into which we are supposed to stick nothing smaller than our elbow (yet often do, despite knowing better). Together, the outer part of the ear and the ear canal serve to gather sound and to direct it deeper into the ear.

The parts of the middle ear are also familiar to most people. They include the eardrum and ear bones (malleus, incus and stapes or hammer, anvil and stirrup if you prefer). The middle ear itself is simply an air-filled space that allows movement of the eardrum and ear bones. The eardrum forms the outermost part of the middle ear. It is connected to the malleus bone which is connected to the incus bone which is connected to the stapes bone. This last bone fits into a small opening (window) between the middle ear and inner ear to transmit sound to the inner ear. The middle ear has to transfer the sound that normally travels through air to the fluids in the inner ear with a minimal loss of power. Simply putting your head under water can demonstrate how much sound can be lost as it passes from air to fluid. The middle ear overcomes this transfer by having the ear bones work in a lever action to transfer the power. The sound power is also preserved by taking all the sound hitting the eardrum and focusing it on the opening to the inner ear (a much smaller space). Once this transfer of sound is accomplished, the middle ear's job is done and it is time for the inner ear to do its thing.

The portion of the inner ear responsible for hearing is called the cochlea (pronounced "Coke" like the soft drink, then "lee" and "ah"). It is outwardly snail shaped and houses the hearing organ (organ of Corti) within its two and one-half turns. Contrary to the popular view, the inner ear does not have just one hearing nerve, but thousands of nerve (hair) cells. As the last little ear bone moves in and out of the window between the middle and inner ear, the fluid in the inner ear is set into motion. The fluid then moves the little hair cells which convert this mechanical energy into electrochemical signals that are sent to the brain. When a person is diagnosed with hearing loss due to nerve damage, the damage is usually in these small hair cells.

11

The other part of the inner ear (the vestibular system) controls balance. Along with vision and feedback from the muscles in the legs, the inner ear helps us detect movement and orient ourselves in three dimensional space. The vestibular system looks something like a roller coaster. There is a main hub from which three canals loop out at differing angles. As in the hearing portion of the inner ear, the vestibular portion works by detecting the motion of fluid. Rather than sound moving the fluid, gravity and the motion of our bodies cause movement. If we go forward, the fluid tries to move back. If we go back, the fluid tries to move forward. Gravity tries to pull the fluid down if we are right side up or towards the top of the head if we are upside down. The vestibular system detects all of this.

Having omitted schematics, diagrams and lots of words derived from foreign languages, this was, of course, not the most detailed description of the ear. However, it should not have been too painful and will be sufficient for the discussions in this book.

Ear Lookers

The first step to examining an ear is to look into it. To do this, some form of ear looker is needed. The most basic of these is called an otoscope (ear scope). Aside from its high price, the otoscope is really just a glorified flashlight. Like a flashlight, it has batteries in the handle, a little light bulb, a glass lens and it lights up stuff. In this case, it lights up the ear canal and eardrum. Unlike a flashlight, the otoscope has a cone shaped portion that goes into the person's ear to straighten out the canal and help hold it open. Using an otoscope, an ear professional can visualize the ear canal, the eardrum, and if they are lucky, a little way through the eardrum. Otoscopes are an indispensable tool for ear professionals.

A more impressive kind of ear looker is a video otoscope. Rather than being a glorified flashlight, the video otoscope is a glorified video camera. Like a regular otoscope it lights up the ear canal and eardrum. However, rather than looking through a tiny eyepiece (lens), an image of the ear is displayed on a television monitor. The view through a regular otoscope may be every bit as good, but people usually prefer the video otoscope because they too can see what the ear looks like inside. Video otoscopes can also take pictures of the eardrum for patient records or to send to other professionals when a referral is needed. Most people consider the video otoscope to be a very worthwhile advance over a conventional otoscope. Now they can see what may or may not be wrong without having to depend entirely on a physician's descriptions.

An operation or diagnosis microscope might be considered the ultimate ear looker. It could also be termed an ear looker plus, because it makes possible doing more than looking. As with an otoscope, the view is good. It can also be magnified to whatever extent needed. With a camera attachment, an operation and diagnosis microscope can additionally display the ear on television like a video otoscope. The advantage of the microscope is that it provides a good view while leaving a physician's hands free to perform medical procedures (remove wax, suctioning infection from an ear, patching an eardrum, etc.). Due to its higher cost, the operation and diagnosis microscope may not be as common as a video otoscope. However, when in-office treatment is needed, this is the looker of choice for most ear doctors.

Regardless of the ear looker used, two things have to be kept in mind. The first is that hearing loss as well as many ear diseases may not be visible. Looking in the ears can let a physician rule out a number of pathologies, but it is usually only the starting point for a more complete evaluation. The second thing to keep in mind is that from the standpoint of diagnosis and treatment, the education and experience of the person behind the ear looker is almost always more important than the particular ear looker used.

How Did That Get In There?

It only stands to reason that if we are going to go to the trouble to look in people's ears, we should not be too surprised at what we might find. There are things that develop on their own and things that people purposely, and sometimes not so purposely, put into the ear. Whatever winds up in the ear, a hearing problem can result if the ear canal becomes completely blocked. For the ear to work properly, sound has to get to the eardrum.

Past some unspecified age, a little bit of hair is one of those things that can be found living happily in or at the entrance to the ear canal. It is more common in men, but can occasionally be seen in women. While failing to perform any profound task, the hair does serve very well to collect one of the other things that develop in the ear - earwax. The situation is much like getting gum stuck in your hair. It doesn't come out. The analogy is visually closer if we think of peanut butter instead of gum. Either way, it is a great big yuck.

Children are by far the most likely to purposely put things into their ears (or the ears of other people who may not be watching them closely). Beads, crayons, rocks and dirt all find their way into children's ears. Assorted vegetables that they would rather not eat also end up in the ears. Parents rarely think to look there! Most of the time parents are unaware their child has anything in the ear unless they don't seem to hear, the ear becomes painful, starts to swell or whatever was planted there begins to grow.

A more distasteful category of things that wind up in the ear, are those that get there on their own power while looking for something good to eat or for a nice place to live. This can apply to a great number of creepy crawly things, but most often applies to cockroaches. One of the little critters can crawl into the ear canal while a person sleeps and then it can't turn around to get out. It just pounds against the eardrum until the person does something about it. Almost too much fun for any one person to have.

Regardless of what got into the ear or how it got there, your doctor is the person to see to get it out. This may be a primary care physician, pediatrician or ear specialist. Whatever is in there, they have likely seen it before and removed worse. Don't be surprised, however, if they ask how it got there. Doctors like a good story.

Send In The Psychics

Some ear problems are physically pretty obvious. It does not take the worlds leading diagnostician to recognize earwax. Similarly, if a person comes to the office with green drainage oozing from the ear and has a history of ear infections, they likely have an ear infection. Aside from ear infections, eardrum perforations and earwax, the majority of ear problems are not visible during a physical exam. The best ear looker in the world won't be enough. Tests are needed.

A hearing test is the simplest and most useful tool for figuring out what is going on with the ears. It has value beyond just indicating the amount of hearing loss. Most ear diseases affect the hearing in some way. A hearing loss caused by noise exposure will have a pattern that is different from a hearing loss caused by aging, infection or various other ear diseases. In this way, the test can give an indication of what is causing the problem. Further, the hearing test also shows where in the ear the problem lies. By finding the location of the problem, the hearing test serves as an important indicator of what can or cannot be done to correct the problem. When the cause of the problem is unclear from the history, physical exam and hearing test, this combination can usually suggest what other tests could be of value.

In our era of skepticism and investigative reporting, most people are concerned about "unnecessary charges." Skepticism regarding the necessity of medical tests often runs rampant, even when a test is specifically requested by a physician. In the case of ear problems, this results in people stating that they do not want a hearing test even before they have described their problem. This leaves them wanting a psychic doctor. They are wishing their doctor to divine the problem without permitting the tools required. It is not necessarily that hearing health care professionals are any less psychic than anyone else. This is not what they are being paid to do. They are being paid to find out what is wrong, not to predict or guess.

The Hearing Test

For many, the thought of a hearing test brings back memories of the school nurse wanting you to raise your hand when there was a sound. For others, the test represents some kind of strange ritual involving a sound proof trailer that mysteriously appears once or twice a year outside of work. Employees are herded out to the trailer, respond to a few beeps and then it is back to work they go. However, for a great many of us, the thought of a hearing test conjures up no memories at all, because we have never had one.

What most people think of as a hearing test (listening to beeps though headphones) is only one part of a complete hearing evaluation. For this most familiar part of the hearing test, the task is to press a button, raise a hand, or respond in some other way whenever there is a beep: even if it sounds very quiet. This shows the lowest level at which a person can hear at a number of different pitches. In settings where the goal is simply to rule out hearing loss (schools, hearing screenings, etc.), this is frequently the only testing that is performed. It is also all that is generally done in industrial settings where the goal is to determine if the hearing is being

16

damaged over time due to noise exposure. The test is performed in a quiet sound proof room with no distractions. This provides a repeatable condition. It also allows the monitoring of changes in hearing over time. It is understood that this represents an ideal, rather than real world listening condition. However, it provides a concrete measure in at least one situation of how an individual hears in comparison to others. By itself, this part of the hearing test is often not medically helpful and is of limited value beyond the examples listed above. It only gives an indication of the softest sounds an individual says they can hear.

A second part of a complete hearing test is to determine how softly a person can hear a series of two syllable words. These words provide a double check to insure that the person responded accurately to the beeps. If a child keeps raising their hand even when they do not hear the beeps, they will not be able to repeat words presented at this same soft level. Similarly, some adults may want to give the appearance of good hearing to pass safety standards for a job or for other reasons. The comparison of hearing levels for tones and words pick up these individuals also. This comparison can additionally be used to detect people exaggerating or faking a hearing loss. Rarely do they get their volunteered thresholds for words and tones to match closely enough not to indicate a problem.

The first two parts of the hearing test are concerned with how soft people can hear. The third part of the test focuses on how clearly a person can hear. To measure this, the person is asked to repeat a series of words that are presented at a volume well above their hearing threshold (the softest level they can hear). The words used for this test are specially selected to represent an even mix of the different speech sounds used in the English language (there are special word lists for other languages also). If a person can repeat all or nearly all of the words, they have good clarity of hearing (also called understanding, discrimination, or word recognition ability). If a person can make out few or none of the words they have very poor or no clarity. The clarity of hearing is in many ways, more important than how soft a person can hear. It is much better to have good word understanding than a good hearing level, because sounds can always be made louder. Sounds can not generally be made clearer. Consequently, reporting the lowest level at which a person can hear is largely useless without also reporting the clarity with which they hear.

Similar to the first part of the hearing test, the last part also uses beeps at a variety of pitches to see how soft a person can hear. The difference is in the headphone. For the first part of the hearing test a conventional headphone is used. The sound goes into the ear canal, moves the eardrum, the little ear bones, the parts of the inner ear and gets sent to the brain so the person can hear. For this last part of the hearing test, a special headphone called a bone vibrator is placed behind the ear. This headphone gently vibrates the skull. Rather than the eardrum, ear bones and other parts of the ear moving, they remain still while the rest of the head moves around them. The result is that the middle ear (ear bones and eardrum) is bypassed and a direct measure of how well the inner ear hears is obtained. If the results from this test and the first one are identical, then we know that no sound is being lost as it goes through the middle ear. If the person hears well on this test but poorly on the first test, we know that the hearing nerve works well but the sound is being blocked by the middle ear. In this last case the hearing loss would be in the middle ear and may be correctable by a physician.

While not high-tech, the four parts of the hearing test combined can be a very powerful tool. They show the amount of hearing loss, indicate where in the ear the hearing problem is, whether the hearing has changed and can often give an indication of the cause. The results can also determine whether a particular hearing loss can be corrected. Since testing equipment is set to a national standard and the same word lists are used from hearing center to hearing center and from year to year, the tests are very repeatable between centers and comparable over time.

Decibels And Percentages

Once the hearing is tested, we have to be concerned with what the results mean. Is there a hearing loss, and if so, how much? How is it quantified?

If asked, many ear doctors, audiologists and hearing aid dealers will look at the test results and quote the amount of hearing loss as a percentage. Doing it this way is technically incorrect and to a certain extent misleading. All ear professionals know this, but sometimes choose to talk in percentages anyway. People understand percentages and are comfortable dealing with them. If hearing loss were explained in a way that was technically correct, more time would likely be spent discussing mathematical concepts than on the hearing loss itself. By expressing the amount of hearing loss as a percentage, the majority of time can be spent discussing the hearing loss and what can be done about it.

For those who want to be technically correct, hearing is measured in decibels (dB). The basic unit for reporting sound levels (the Bel) was named for Alexander Graham Bell. When measuring hearing, the decibel (1/10 Bel) is used. The range is 0 dB for the softest sounds people can hear, up to 140 dB for sounds that are so loud as to be very painful and potentially destructive. Contrary to expectations, a sound that is 140 dB is not 100 or 140 times greater than a sound that is 0 dB. It is 10,000,000 times greater. To make matters worse, decibels are not measured on a linear scale, they are measured on a logarithmic one. This means that the actual sound pressure level grows at a faster and faster rate as we move from 0 dB up the scale. The sound pressure level at 20 dB represents a 10 fold increase over the sound pressure level at 0 dB. The sound pressure level at 40 dB represents a 100 fold increase over the sound pressure level at 0 dB. Sixty dB is a 1,000 fold increase, 80 dB a 10,000 fold increase, etc. All of this is then plotted on a graph called an audiogram. The graph shows how powerful (loud) different pitched sounds have to become before a person can hear them. This system makes perfect sense to ear professionals and to the few non-mathematicians who routinely think in logarithmic terms. It is less than intuitive for the rest of us. It would be nice if we could use a linear scale, but the ear does not work that way.

So, when ear doctors, audiologists and hearing aid dealers talk about the percentage of hearing loss, what are they talking about? Usually, it is how loud sounds have to become before they are heard (30 dB, 40 dB, 50 dB etc.). They take the decibel level and call it a percentage. This works fairly well because most people do not care about the physics of sound and because people who cannot hear sounds at 100 dB (i.e. a 100% loss) appear pretty much deaf anyway. Hearing professionals may additionally classify a hearing loss as mild (hearing thresholds in the 20-40 dB range), moderate (40-60 dB), moderately-severe (60-80 dB), severe (80-100 dB) or profound (>100 dB).There are more exotic percentage calculations used to judge disability, liability or hearing handicap, but these are also just simplifications for those who do not like to live in a logarithmic world.

Adventures In Word Misunderstanding

As previously mentioned, some hearing losses may cause the ears to garble or distort words. No matter how clearly or how loudly the words are spoken, the ears will mess up some of them. Given an unclear signal, the brain compensates by filling in what was misunderstood. Sometimes this works well, sometimes not. This is why it is important to look at the clarity of hearing in addition to the level of hearing.

At times the ears mess up words so badly that there is no doubt they were misunderstood. Try as it might, the brain can only respond with a resounding "huh?". Although annoying, an individual knows they missed what was said and can always ask the person to repeat. More problematic are the times when an individual does not realize that they misunderstood what was said. One way or another, the brain fills in the gaps often changing the direction of a conversation from the mundane into high adventure.

Everyone occasionally misunderstands what is said. The results of this are sometimes humorous and at other times embarrassing. People with certain hearing losses can have this happen on a regular basis. They either misunderstand what was said, making them think the person speaking is nuts, or respond inappropriately, making other people think they are nuts. Most of us have a friend or relative that to one degree or another lives this adventure. Many of these people do well by accepting their difficulties with a little humor. Others may dwell on the problem or deny it entirely by placing the blame on others.

One of my more memorable adventures with word misunderstanding involved a hearing impaired nun. She did not think she had much of a hearing problem, but came in for a routine evaluation anyway. As part of the evaluation, she had to repeat a number of tape recorded words in order to determine how good or bad her word understanding might be. The tape contained a nationally standardized list of unremarkable one syllable words such as ran, toy, shoe and ear. When she repeated the first word as "damn" instead of "ran", I suspected that an adventure might be beginning. After repeating (or trying to repeat) the full 50 words, she chastised me at length for forcing her to repeat all those dirty words. Having missed the actual words, she must have concluded that I would be just the sort to have dirty word tapes. Afterwards, I explained that the tapes had ordinary (not dirty) words and that she had misunderstood. However, I think she just figured that it would be in character for anyone who would make a nun repeat lists of dirty words, to also lie about it.

Sounds That Are Not So Sweet

When people lose hearing, sometimes more is lost than the ability to hear soft sounds or clearly understand words. Quite often, they lose some of their ability to distinguish one pitch from another. This is different from someone who is considered "tone deaf" because they cannot sing or hum a particular tone. A person with hearing loss may not be able to hear the difference between tones.

Almost anyone who develops a hearing loss may have difficulty appreciating or enjoying music the way they used to. Sounds can seem discordant or monotone. A person with normal hearing can discriminate almost an infinite number of pitch differences. Musical subtleties are not lost on them. People with hearing loss may discriminate fewer pitches often reducing the depth and beauty of the sound. It is like taking the eighty-eight keys on a piano keyboard and gluing them together in pairs so there are effectively only forty-four keys. It would not sound too good. With a really bad hearing loss, more keys would be glued together making things sound even more discordant.

Even worse, problems with hearing pitch can also affect the ability to understand speech and to distinguish who is speaking. Different speech sounds may not sound different. This can be especially true when people are speaking fast or with a foreign accent. In a group, problems discriminating between different pitches can make it more difficult to focus on just one person. Other people may not sound distinctly different from the person one is trying to hear. When answering the phone, it may be more difficult to immediately recognize who is calling. People start to sound alike. It may become necessary to focus on what is being said, rather than on the voice of the person saying it, to determine who is speaking.

Using a hearing aid can often highlight the problems caused by the inability to differentiate one pitch from another. The hearing aid makes sounds loud enough for the person to hear, but they may not seem clear or natural. Most people's first instinct is to blame the hearing aid for not amplifying the sound clearly. Unfortunately, more often than not, the hearing aid is working fine and it is the person's ear that is not processing the sounds clearly or naturally. Prior to hearing aid use, they did not hear enough of the sound to be aware that the ear was blurring the pitches together. Consequently, a hearing aid may still be useful, but it may not sound perfectly natural since there are fewer keys on the ear's keyboard.

What You Should Hear

All of the testing aside, a person with normal hearing should be able to hear the things that other people hear. Someone with a hearing loss does less well. If a person does only slightly worse, this may be a normal variation from person to person. But, if they do much worse, it is likely a hearing loss. If the rest of the audience at a theater or movie can hear and understand the actors, then you should too if your hearing is normal. If your family can hear and understand Aunt Jane, then you should also. There are an infinite number of sounds. Some of these will be heard, others will not. A hearing problem is only indicated when others consistently hear the things that you do not.

Over the years, many people have been tested to determine what normal hearing is. The majority of tests determine either how soft or how clearly a person can hear. As with other human abilities, there is a range of hearing that is considered normal. Some people will naturally hear a little better or a little worse than others, but overall, people hear about the same. Surprisingly, what may appear or sound natural to an individual is often of little value in assessing hearing ability. It is often more a reflection of what a person is used to, rather than an indication of what the human ear should hear.

What a person should be able to hear will vary depending on the setting. It will be much easier to hear in a quiet room with good acoustics than in a noisy room with poor acoustics. Hearing and understanding a friend in a library will be easier than in an auto plant with the assembly line running. Similarly, hearing in a restaurant will be more difficult when it is busy than in the off-hours. What others can hear in each setting remains an individual's standard of what they should be able to hear in these settings.

While focusing on the places where people are known to have difficulty hearing may be an excellent marketing tool for hearing aids, it does not necessarily help determine whether or not a person has a hearing loss. Since everyone has more difficulty hearing in a background of noise, it does little good to ask a person if they have difficulty hearing in noise. What needs to be asked is whether family or friends hear things in these situations better than you do.

Many will be disappointed that there is no overall list of things a person should or should not be able to hear. What a person should be able to hear at any particular time varies by a such frighteningly complex set of variables that any overall list would likely be wrong most of the time. The measure that remains is how an individual hears in each of these situations in relation to their peers. It may not be as satisfying as a concrete list, but it will more often be a better guide.

Minimal Hearing Loss

Bridging the gap between normal hearing and a noticeable hearing loss is a gray area we might call a minimal hearing loss. This could be defined as hearing that is near-normal, but not quite perfect. Hearing can range from borderline normal up to about a 25% or 30% hearing loss. Minimal hearing loss could also be defined as a hearing loss that is measurable, but has limited or no perceived impact upon a person's activities or lifestyle. However, some would say that no hearing loss is minimal, regardless of how small or whether it was perceived or considered a problem by the person. They might even object to the term "minimal" as trivializing hearing loss.

Ear doctors in hospitals or private practice spend their days seeing people with severe hearing losses, dead (non-hearing) ears, acute infections and all kinds of other nasty ear problems. People come to an ear doctor because they are having problems. The worse the problem, the more likely they are to see a doctor. Those with minimal hearing losses are often the better off people in this setting.

Audiologists and speech pathologists working in schools are much more likely to consider children with minimal hearing losses as the worse off in their settings. The majority of the kids they see are normal. When they find a child with even a small hearing loss, they can seem to stick out like a sore thumb. These few children are viewed as the unlucky ones.

Some people consider their minimal hearing loss to be a non-issue. They may know from testing that a small loss exists or constantly be reminded by friends or relatives that they might have a problem. However, they feel they hear OK in most situations and want to leave well enough alone. Other people may see their minimal hearing loss as a big issue. They can no longer hear everything they need or want to hear and it is having an impact on their lifestyle or relationships. Not only does this small hearing loss bother them, it motivates them to do something about it. They do not care that others might classify their hearing loss as being no big deal, they want it fixed.

One's peer group also serves to determine how a minimal hearing loss will be viewed. A 95 year old person with a 30%

hearing loss would likely be considered to hear well when compared against their 90 something year old peers. Even though they do not hear as well as when they were teenagers, they may hear as well as everyone else in their retirement home. However, if we give this same 30% hearing loss to a third grade student, it will put them at a distinct disadvantage to their peers. As they fall behind their classmates, the hearing loss may not appear so "minimal".

A minimal hearing loss may not be large enough to cause a problem for everyone, but for a person who needs to hear well, it can be devastating. Recognizing those people significantly affected by a minimal loss from those not significantly affected, is the primary consideration about how to proceed. If the hearing loss (no matter how small) causes a person a significant problem, it should be corrected to the greatest extent possible. If the hearing loss does not cause much of a problem, it is often possible for a person to live their life and not worry about it too much.

One final point that needs to be understood in this discussion is that a minimal hearing loss is still a hearing loss. The cause needs to be identified in order to be sure it is not something that requires medical treatment. A minimal hearing loss might only be the first sign of something more serious or of a hearing loss that could progress if untreated.

Types Of Hearing Loss

Once we have found a hearing loss and quantified it in some way, we need to find out what type of hearing loss it is in order to determine what can be done about it. Hearing loss is generally divided into three major types based on where in the ear the problem lies. These types are different from a diagnosis. They do not classify the amount of hearing loss or its underlying cause. They simply point to the location of the problem.

The first type is termed a conductive hearing loss. If the loss is due to a problem with the outer ear, ear canal, eardrum or ear bones, the loss is termed conductive. If something prevents any of these structures from doing their job, this kind of hearing loss results. The sound is not transferred (conducted) efficiently to the inner ear. An ear infection, earwax, a hole in the eardrum or a broken ear bone are a few of the possible causes for a conductive hearing loss. Many conductive hearing losses can be lessened or medically corrected. Earwax can be removed, an ear infection cured, a torn eardrum patched and a broken ear bone replaced. Not all conductive losses can be corrected, but many can. A person with a conductive hearing loss should never consider hearing aids unless they have first seen an ear doctor to make sure that the loss cannot be corrected.

The second type of hearing loss is termed sensorineural. This is what most people refer to as a nerve hearing loss. The damage is to the little hair (nerve) cells in the inner ear and is not usually medically correctable. However, hearing aids may be used to help compensate for the hearing loss. Even though a nerve hearing loss is not usually correctable, it is important to find out the cause to minimize or prevent further loss of hearing.

The third kind of hearing loss (mixed) is the combination of a conductive and a nerve hearing loss in the same ear. By definition, a person cannot have both a conductive and a nerve hearing loss in the same ear. They have a mixed hearing loss which is, of course, both a conductive and nerve hearing loss. Although defined as one type of hearing loss, treatment for the nerve and conductive parts of a mixed loss have to be addressed separately.

Now that the three major kinds of hearing loss have been described, we will mention a fourth and fifth that are much less common. The first of these is called a retrocochlear hearing loss. This is any hearing loss that results from damage or malformation beyond the inner ear. It could be a problem

27

with the nerve that carries sound from the inner ear to the brain or a problem with how the brain itself processes the sound. In either case, the ear works well to pick up and process sound. The sound is messed up somewhere further down the line.

The final type of hearing loss is not real. This is termed a non-organic hearing loss. A person faking a hearing loss appears to all the world as hearing impaired despite having no ear problem. Similarly, it is possible for psychological problems to interfere with the proper recognition of sounds processed by the ears. In either case, there is a "functional" (another name for a non-organic loss) hearing loss in that people do not respond to sounds appropriately. Fortunately, this kind of inappropriate response to sound is fairly easy to detect and separate from a hearing loss originating in the ear itself.

In order to determine whether a hearing loss might be treatable, it is necessary to localize where in the ear the problem lies. Classifying hearing loss into these types gives hearing professionals a shorthand method for identifying the location of the damage or disease. Diagnosis of the cause and treatment can proceed from there. Discussion of the individual diseases that can produce these types of hearing loss are provided in chapter five.

Noise Induced Hearing Loss

Of all of the types of hearing loss, the most preventable is a noise induced hearing loss. This is simply a sensorineural (nerve) loss that has been caused by extremely loud or repeated exposure to loud noise. Aside from infection and disease, loud noise poses the greatest danger to a person's hearing. Those who work in loud noise or participate in very loud activities or hobbies, are the ones at risk. Sounds can become so loud that their force (sound pressure) can literally tear the little nerve cells in the inner ear. The nerves cannot repair themselves or regrow. Permanent hearing loss results. The damage builds up gradually following months and years of noise exposure. A few of the little hearing nerves are damaged one day, a few more the next and pretty soon the numbers start to add up. Life in the inner ear begins to resemble the set for an apocalyptic movie.

Given enough exposure, many sounds can be loud enough to cause at least some hearing loss. A partial list of potential offenders might include power tools, construction equipment, lawn mowers, leaf blowers, gasoline powered trimmers, chain saws, snowmobiles, motorcycles, outboard motors, sirens, fireworks, firearms, rock concerts, auto races, stereo equipment and some children's toys. The workplace can also provide a variety of destructive sounds. Few would be surprised that the sounds in a metal stamping plant would be loud enough to damage the ears. But how many would think that a band director or a toll booth operator on the turnpike might be at risk?

Fortunately, regulations do exist to protect us from loud noise in the workplace. Ear protection (ear plugs or muffs) is required in all settings where sound pressure levels have been found to be at potentially dangerous levels. People exposed to varying levels of noise throughout the workday may be required to occasionally wear a device that measures their total daily exposure of noise. If the total exposure is found to be at a dangerous level, the person would be required to wear ear protection during more of their workday. Regulations also require companies to test employees' hearing annually if they are being exposed to loud noise. If the hearing is found to change as a result of noise exposure, the employee might be required to wear more effective ear protection, use both earplugs and earmuffs, or they might be moved to a quieter job where there is a lessened risk of hearing damage.

Failure to wear earplugs or earmuffs is the primary cause for preventable work related hearing losses. Although employees have been told that their work areas are loud enough to cause hearing loss, some still do not wear the ear protection provided. They might not like the way the earplugs or muffs feel or the inconvenience of them. They may believe they are too macho or do not need to wear them. Often the complaint is that the plugs or muffs make it too difficult to hear their machine or co-workers well. But if they do not wear them, in a few years they may not be able to hear their machine or co-workers, even without earplugs. Years ago, people worked long hours in loud noise and ended up with huge hearing losses. They didn't know that the noise could be damaging, and industry at the time was not required to provide any protection. Things are different today. Many of the workers currently developing noise induced hearing losses are choosing to do so by not wearing their ear protection. Unlike their predecessors, they know the noise can cause hearing loss, and they know how to prevent it. They just don't act on it. They probably don't wear their seat belts either.

While big brother may be looking over our shoulder at work to keep us hearing, there are no ear police at home. We can shoot ten thousand rounds of ammunition every year or play the stereo so loud that the floor gives us a massage. We can sit in the front row at rock concerts or use power tools all day. No one will come into our house to measure how loud the sounds are or whether they might be dangerous. We are on our own. As a general rule, the sound should be considered too loud if it makes the ears feel full, hurt or ring, or if you or someone else must shout to be heard over the noise. If this happens, turning down the volume, wearing earplugs or spending less time exposed to loud sounds, would be in order.

The most convenient sources for earplugs and earmuffs are hardware stores, home improvement centers and gun stores. The hardware and home improvement stores sell them for use with power tools. Gun shops sell them to protect the hearing while shooting. Most earplugs and muffs reduce the overall volume by about 25 or 30%. This is enough for most purposes. If more protection is needed, earplugs and muffs can be worn together. This over-the-counter protection works well for the majority. For people who require hearing protection but still need to hear very well regardless of earplugs or earmuffs, there are more personal and exotic options. An example would be musician's earplugs which are specially designed to reduce all of the pitches equally so that the most natural sound possible is maintained. Another would be electronic earmuffs that transmit all but loud sounds into the ears. An audiologist or hearing aid dealer would be able to provide more information on these and other options for hearing protection.

People working or playing in loud noise really have very little choice about wearing or not wearing something in or over their ears. The only choice they have is whether it will be earplugs or muffs now, or hearing aids later.

Car Stereos

Car stereos can be unexpected sources of noise induced hearing loss. Stereos have become standard equipment on most cars, trucks and vans. At worst, we consider them as background noise or an unneeded gadget. More often they serve as entertainment or as a companion to keep us awake on a long drive. The majority of us would not consider buying a car without a stereo. We can get ones that will play cassettes, CDs, or ones with graphic equalizers allowing us to tinker with the sound in a great number of ways. Most of these stereos have lots of neat knobs and buttons that are fun to push and we routinely do so with little thought or recognition of any possible harm.

While we may not think of the typical car stereo as being very loud, it has to be loud enough to get above the road, engine, wind, rain and other environmental noises. To hear the stereo clearly over these noises, some of us may adjust the volume loud enough to cause hearing loss. The area inside a car can be uniquely dangerous to our ears because it is a small enclosed space. This can be wonderful for the sound quality, but terrible for our ears. Since the sound has nowhere to dissipate, the sound pressure can build to levels that may actually tear the little nerve cells in the inner ear. The situation is not unlike sitting inside a bass drum while someone outside is pounding on it. The sound would be very clear and realistic, but probably not too comfortable. Fortunately, most people do not turn their car stereos up to these dangerous levels, or they turn them down if the sound becomes uncomfortably loud. This is a matter of common sense and works for most people.

The above applies to normal people with normal car stereos. However, there are car stereos that are much louder than normal, greatly increasing the risk of damage to our ears. These are generally not the ones that come as standard equipment. They are usually added later by teenagers specifically for their loudness (teenagers usual belief that they are immortal also applies to their ears). It is easy to recognize cars equipped with these sound systems by their ability to vibrate surrounding cars, busses, houses, businesses, public structures and unsuspecting farm animals as they drive by. There are actually contests for these loud stereos in which the systems are judged for absolute loudness or clarity of sound. The contestants turn on and adjust their stereos from outside the vehicle by remote control. Spectators listen from bleachers that are placed a safe distance away. Everyone has the good sense not to sit in the vehicle while all this is happening. Full-on, some of these systems can blow the windows right out of a car. Imagine what they could do to your ears.

A Hearing Loss Is A Hearing Loss

A common mistake is to think that all hearing losses are the same. While this view may not necessary qualify someone as a bad person, it is a stereotype. Someone knowing a hearing impaired person may assume that all other hearing impaired people are just like them. If the known person has a horrible hearing loss and does poorly even with hearing aids, the stereotype might be that hearing impaired people cannot function well in society or that hearing aids do not work. If the hearing impaired person had their hearing restored through surgery, then the stereotype might be that all hearing losses can be corrected, or that one particular surgeon can correct all hearing losses. Like the majority of stereotypes, hearing loss stereotypes are most often wrong when applied to anyone beyond the individual on which they are based.

People with differing amounts of hearing loss have differing amounts of handicap. In general, people with milder hearing losses do better than people with larger losses. People with better word understanding do better than people with poorer word understanding. How a person does can also vary depending on which pitches the person does not hear well (high pitches vs. low pitches, etc.). With all the combinations of hearing ability that can be obtained by mixing these three variables (hearing level, clarity and pitch of hearing loss), it is not surprising that all of the hearing impaired will not perform the same.

In addition, the way we view the consequences of a hearing loss has to include not just what a person can hear, but what the person needs to hear to do their job or live their life. A child in school needs to hear just about everything, while a retired or semi-retired person sitting on their front porch may not need to hear a great deal. A fairly large hearing loss might not greatly affect the person sitting on the porch while a very small hearing loss might cause the child to fail in school. Consequently, we must take into account everything a person has to do, needs to do or may want to do, to have any idea of how a particular hearing loss will affect them. This being the case, it can be difficult to predict how even one hearing impaired person will do in most situations. Obviously, a single prediction (stereotype) applied to all hearing impaired people would be wrong.

What You May Not Want To Hear

Now comes the real horror of ear mechanics. What many have suspected but were too cautious or afraid to confront is indeed true. Those who are squeamish or without the most serious resolve to recognize and embrace a potentially unsettling ear truth, may wish to proceed no further. Stop now.

If still reading, we will assume you have thrown caution to the wind or have a deep desire to know. While it may be difficult to anticipate what might instill this profound dread, deep down, you may suspect or possibly know.

The way you sound to yourself is not the way others hear you! The way you sound on tape is actually the way you sound!

This horror of ear mechanics results from hearing yourself speak in a physically different way from which you hear others. When another speaks, the sound leaves their mouth, travels through the air and hits your eardrum. The eardrum is moved as well as the little bones in the middle ear. The last of the little ear bones moves in and out of a small opening in the inner ear causing the fluid in the inner ear to move. As the fluid in the inner ear moves, the little hair (nerve) cells react by turning this mechanical motion into electro-chemical signals which are sent to the brain. Then you hear. The sound is connected to the eardrum which is connected to the ear bones which is connected to the inner ear which is connected to your brain.

When you hear yourself talking, it doesn't work quite that way. Rather than the sound leaving your mouth, wandering into your ear and moving the eardrum, something a little

34

more direct is involved. As a person talks, the vibrations from their own vocal cords set their skull into vibration. Instead of going to the trouble to shake the eardrum, ear bones and parts of the inner ear, nature largely leaves these parts alone and shakes the head instead. People hear by the relative movement of the inner parts of the ear in relation to the head. It doesn't matter whether the inner parts of the ear move and the head remains still or whether the head moves and the inner parts of the ear remain still. Either way, you hear.

The reason these two conditions sound different is that in the case of your own voice, the resonance of your skull shapes the sound. The situation is analogous to the sounding board of a piano. The vibration of the wood in the piano provides a richer and more pleasing sound than would be created by the vibration of the strings alone. Similarly, it is the vibration of our own skulls that makes the perception of our own voice richer and more pleasing than when we hear ourselves on tape.

Trivia

No discussion of hearing basics would be complete without at least some trivia. Below are a few items to fill this need.

1. The best known piece of ear trivia is that the smallest bones in the human body are the three middle ear bones. In fact, they are so small that all three can fit on the face of a dime with room to spare. The smallest (the stapes) is only a few millimeters across at its widest point. The other two middle ear bones (the malleus and incus) are a little bit bigger, but not much. When trivia games or contests ask a question about the ear, nine times out of ten they want to know the name of the smallest ear bone or where it is in the body.

2. Most people are somewhat aware that a normal hearing person can detect sounds over a range of 20 - 20,000 cycles / second (cps). Each cycle can be thought of as one complete

ocean wave. However, rather than the waves being made of water and moving across the surface of the ocean, they are sound waves moving through the air. A very low pitched sound would have few of these waves hitting the eardrum each second. A high pitched sound would have thousands of waves hitting the eardrum each second. What is not commonly understood is that the ear is not equally sensitive to all of these pitches. A normal ear will be able to detect very weak sounds in the middle pitches, while at the extreme low or high pitches, the sound pressure level may need to be as much as 10,000 times greater to be heard. If we go back to our ocean analogy, little ripples in the water would be easily detectable if they were at the ear's preferred pitches (1000 - 3000 cps). At the extreme high or low frequencies, a tidal wave might go by unnoticed. This is why very high or low pitched sounds are more likely than middle pitched sounds to be perceived as annoying or uncomfortably loud. Even when they may not sound very loud, the sound pressure level is much greater and can even be painful.

3. Another bit of pitch related trivia has to do with how we perceive different pitched sounds. Since the pitches we hear range from 20 - 20,000 cps, we might expect the center of this range (about 10,000 cps) to sound like a middle pitched sound. In reality, it is perceived as an extremely high pitched sound. Perceptually, the center most pitch in our hearing range is about 640 cps (middle C on a piano keyboard is 256 cps). This happens because our 20,000 cps pitch range is perceived over 10 octaves. The first octave is 20 - 40 cps, the second 40 - 80 cps, the third 80 - 160 cps, the fourth 160 - 320 cps, the fifth 320 - 640 cps, the sixth 640 - 1280 cps, the seventh 1280 - 2560 cps, the eighth 2560 - 5120 cps, the ninth 5120 - 10,240 cps and the tenth 10,240 - 20,480 cps. Despite each octave's different frequency size, each is perceived as the equivalent of eight notes on a piano keyboard. The 20 - 40 cps range and the 10,240 - 20,480 cps range each have eight notes. Consequently, if a person lost all

36

of their hearing above 10,000 cps, they would only lose one octave: not half their hearing.

4. This final piece of trivia has more to do with physics than the ear, but we will include it anyway since hearing is involved. We all know that light travels faster than sound. The speed of light is 186,000 miles / second, while the speed of sound through air is a much slower 1130 feet / second. This difference can result in our seeing things that are some distance away before we hear any sound associated with them. We will see lightning flash and then hear it. We will see the flash from sky rockets and then hear them explode. The further away we are, the greater the lag between the two. Of interest here, is that the length of this lag between seeing and hearing something can be used to determine how far away it is. Since light travels very fast, we are usually seeing things at the instant they happen (even if we are seeing them from miles away). On the other hand, it takes sound about five seconds to travel a mile. So, if we see lightning flash and don't hear the boom for five seconds, we know it was about one mile away. If we don't hear the boom for 10 seconds, it was two miles away, 15 seconds was three miles away and so on and so forth. If you see a storm coming and want to know how far away it is, watch for a flash of lightning and then count.

We could easily include many other useful and not so useful items of hearing trivia. However, we will leave the reader to pick out their own favorites from the rest of the book.

Chapter Two: Common Concerns

Ear Wax

Ear wax (cerumen) is a substance that needs little description. It is generally brownish in color, hard if dry, sticky when wet and tastes bad. Most people have some and no one is overly thrilled about it. The most common questions regarding ear wax are: Why is it there? What should I do about it?

There is not total agreement as to the purpose of ear wax. The evolutionary point of view is that ear wax serves some important (even if undiscovered) function. Some believe the purpose is to lubricate the ear canal, but it is yet to be explained why the ear canal needs lubricated any more than the parts of the body which are forced to exist without this substance. A more popular view is that ear wax serves a protective function. An insect or spider that might want to make a home in the human ear quickly becomes so disgusted with this sticky foul tasting stuff that it leaves in search of a place where this kind of thing doesn't happen.

Regardless of its purpose, for most people, the best thing to do with ear wax is leave it alone. The wax tends to work its way out on its own and does not usually need to be cleaned from the ear canals. Wiping the outer part of the ears with a washcloth is generally enough. The use of bobby pins or cotton swabs in the ear canal may push the wax further into the ear, sometimes even packing it up against the eardrum. Also, putting objects into the ear can be dangerous. Accidents can and do happen. One good bump or sneeze while cleaning the ear and there becomes more to worry about than ear wax. Some physicians feel that cotton swabs are useful for cleaning wax at the outer part of the ear canal, but others recommend avoiding their use altogether.

For a small number of people, the ear wax can naturally build up to a point that it completely blocks the ear canal. The presence of this much wax is often accompanied by a plugged feeling and hearing loss. Sometimes, there will also be a ringing or roaring sound (tinnitus) in the ear. Once the ear wax is removed, these symptoms should disappear (provided the wax was the cause).

Several options are available if the amount of ear wax reaches a point that it needs to be removed. The first option is to have the wax removed by a professional. This could include ear doctors, primary care doctors, nurses, audiologists or other health care professionals depending on their training and the equipment available. The wax might be washed, curetted, suctioned or pulled from the ear depending on which appears most appropriate. People with recurring wax problems could have this done periodically (every few months, once a year, twice a year or as needed). No other care would be required.

For the do-it-yourself types, it is possible to remove wax from your ears at home. There are a number of over-the-counter ear washes that can be very effective when used as directed. The major drawback to some of these washes is that they can sometimes irritate the ear canal and should not be used if there is a hole in the eardrum. Washing the ears with peroxide can have the same drawbacks. Consequently, these washes may be best indicated for people who have had a recent physical or ear exam and know that their eardrums are intact. In the cases where it is not known whether there might be a hole in the eardrum, there are eardrops and washes that can be recommended by your doctor that can be used even when there is a hole in the eardrum. Never use old eardrops or washes that are beyond their expiration date.

In brief, while ear wax is fairly common, it is not a problem for the majority of people. For the few individuals in which it does become a problem, the wax can be removed simply and safely in the office by a health care professional or an appropriate at-home treatment can be recommend.

Tinnitus

Tinnitus is a subjective ringing, roaring, chirping, hissing, sea shell or rushing sound in the ears. Each person with tinnitus is likely to describe it a little differently, but all agree that it can be annoying. The sounds are described as soft by some and louder by others. Usually tinnitus is more noticeable at night or when a person is in a quiet place where there are few outside sounds to cover it up. The most common questions regarding tinnitus are the same ones people ask about earwax. Why is it there? What can I do about it?

Tinnitus is not a disease. Rather, it is most often a symptom of blockage or damage in the ear. Tinnitus does not prevent a person from hearing and will not cause a person to go deaf. When the underlying cause is something that can be medically or surgically treated, the tinnitus is often reduced or eliminated following treatment. Seeing an ear doctor or audiologist is the first step to identifying the cause or to rule out any potentially nasty stuff.

When there is nerve damage in the inner ear, tinnitus is very common. Unlike other areas of the body, there are no pain sensors in the inner ear. Damage here is perceived as sound. For example, if a person were unfortunate or stupid enough to take a hammer and smash the fingers of their opposite hand, it would likely hurt. The damaged nerves in the fingers would send a message to the brain and the person would say ouch (or something more graphic). When there is damage in the inner ear, the nerves also send a message to the brain, but it is heard rather than felt. The little nerves in the inner ear sing up a storm and the person has to listen to them. It does not matter whether the damage was caused by disease, trauma, noise exposure or some other agent. The nerves still sing about it.

Almost everyone will experience at least some tinnitus if you can get them in a quiet enough place. By reducing the outside sounds to a low enough level, they can then hear their own head noises. Anything that blocks the ears or prevents outside sounds from being heard can produce this effect. Most hearing losses will increase a person's chance of experiencing tinnitus. If a person has wax or infection that blocks the ears, they will also end up hearing their own head noises. Removing the wax or eliminating the infection usually takes care of the problem. Similarly, if a person's tinnitus is due to a perforated eardrum or damaged ear bones not transmitting sound properly, the tinnitus is often reduced or eliminated by surgically repairing the eardrum or ear bones. If it is possible to fix the ear problem or hearing loss, it is often possible to overcome any associated tinnitus.

Unfortunately, in the majority of cases, it is not possible to correct the underlying cause of the tinnitus. For these people, the options are to live with the head noises, use other sounds to cover them up, or try medications which may lessen the severity of the problem. The majority of people get used to or just learn to live with it. The tinnitus usually becomes less annoying as time passes. People come to realize they are not going to explode or die because of it. Those with hearing aids often find that being able to hear the outside world again also means that their tinnitus gets covered up. People with normal hearing can use a radio, television, fan or other noise sources to produce the same result. Medications are available which may reduce the severity of tinnitus, but these are usually reserved for more severe cases. There are also alternative therapies and support groups for tinnitus. An ear doctor or audiologist would be able to provide information if these are needed.

Pressure

At one time or another, most people have experienced a feeling of fullness or pressure in their ears. They may wonder why this sensation occurs or whether it should cause concern.

If the sensation of pressure comes and goes, it is most likely due to an occasional imbalance between the air pressure inside the middle ear and the air pressure outside the ear. A slight reduction in hearing may accompany this. The pressure imbalance is most likely to be noted while driving in the mountains or while traveling in a pressurized airplane. As the pressure outside the body changes, it takes the ears a little bit of time to adapt and equalize the pressure. When the pressure does equalize, the ears will sometimes seem to "pop". The plugged sensation will go away and the hearing will improve.

The eustachian tube (one for each ear) is responsible for keeping the pressure inside the middle ear equal to the pressure outside the ear. It leads from the back of the throat up and outward to the middle ear. The eustachian tube opens naturally as we chew, swallow, yawn and do a number of other things. It lets air into the ear if more is needed or out of the ear if there is too much. The majority of the time, the eustachian tubes do their job unnoticed.

If the pressure in the middle ear does become less than or greater than the pressure outside the ear, the eardrum will be sucked back or will bulge out because of the pressure imbalance. If the pressure imbalance becomes great enough, it can be very painful as the eardrum and surrounding tissues are stretched to their limit. The hearing may be affected a little bit by the pressure stiffening the eardrum so that it can't move well. Anything that irritates the back of the throat (colds, allergies, smoking, etc.) can make it more difficult for the eustachian tube to open and do its job.

A person can help the eustachian tube to equalize the pressure in a number of ways. One of the simplest is chewing gum. This has been a long time folk remedy to prevent ear pain while driving in the mountains or flying in a plane. If the pressure in the middle ear is less than normal (as often happens to people with a cold due to swelling of the eustachian tube decreasing airflow into the middle ear), air can manually be forced back into the ears. One can take a deep breath, close their mouth, hold the end of the nose closed and then blow like they are blowing their nose. Since there is nowhere else for the air to go, some of it will be forced up into the ear. If the pressure in the middle ear is too much as can occasionally happen with repeated nose blowing, then a person can suck air back out of their ears. This can be done by closing the mouth, holding the nose and swallowing. Another way would be to hold the nose and drink a glass of water.

Aside from these age old remedies to relieve a pressure imbalance within the ear, there is a new remedy or preventative specifically for people who fly. This involves wearing a special set of earplugs during the flight. The earplugs smooth out any rapid pressure changes within the plane so that the ears have more time to adjust.

If the ears always feel full or under pressure, see your doctor. This could indicate a problem that needs to be addressed. If the feeling of pressure is only occasional and clears up by itself, it is most likely normal ear stuff and not a problem.

Common Experiences

There are a number of other common ear related phenomena that people notice or become concerned about. These reports often take the classic form of, "but doctor when I do this, so and so happens". Some of the reports are rather creative, leaving one to wonder what ever caused the person to do their particular "this" in the first place. Others are very common.

Probably the most common phenomenon patients report is how much better they hear when they cup a hand behind their ear. This turns out to be true for everyone. The hand funnels additional sound into the ear that would otherwise just pass on by. The outer part of the ear is shaped so that it naturally acts to direct some sound into the ear. Adding a hand to the ear only increases this effect. Prior to the advances in electronics which made hearing aids possible, collecting additional sound and funneling it into the ear was the only way to hear better. People would use an ear horn with a big opening at one end to collect as much sound as possible and a small opening at the other end that fit into the ear. The sound would get louder as it was squeezed into the smaller and smaller space near the earpiece. It was not a very inconspicuous device (looking like the top of an old style phonograph), but neither is holding a hand behind your ear.

Another common experience is ear pain when a person smiles, frowns or holds their mouth a certain way. Rather than being an ear problem, this is often the result of the jaw joint binding or not moving as it should. Due to some peculiarities of human anatomy, this pain is often felt in the ear rather than in the jaw. A full ear examination is the first step. If the ear exam is negative, then the next step is to see a dentist. When the pain is due to a problem with the jaw joint, the dentist can recommend steps to treat it. Once the problem with the jaw joint is addressed, the ear pain usually goes away.

As a general rule, if something you're doing helps you to hear and you don't look too odd doing it, go for it. On the other hand, if something you are doing is making it more difficult to hear or is causing pain or dizziness, don't do that. Instead, call your doctor and tell them what happens when you do what you do. They might just be able to make it stop doing that.

Background Noise

Whenever hearing difficulties are discussed, it is never long before the issue of background noise is brought up. Background noise could be described as any sound that we do not wish to focus on at the moment. In a car, road and wind sounds are background noise. The radio would be background noise if we are trying to hear a passenger, or the passenger would be background noise if we are trying to hear the radio. Both the radio and passenger could be background noise if we are trying to identify a strange sound the car is making. In and around the home, there are a variety of other sounds that might be considered as background noise. A short list might include the refrigerator, microwave, blender, dishwasher, clothes washer, dryer, vacuum cleaner, fans, furnace, television, radio, lawn mower, floors or hinges squeaking, doors closing, toilets flushing, water running, etc. However, if we want to hear any of these, they would not be background noise. As in the car, we might want to listen to other people in the house or we may consider them as more noise. We live in a world of sound, but these sounds do not become background noise until we decide we are not interested in them or do not want to hear them.

The majority of us do well sorting out the things we wish to listen to, from those things we do not. However, this does not mean that we hear everything we want or that some sounds do not cover up others. Obviously, it would not be possible to hear birds chirping while standing next to a fire siren. Similarly, it becomes more difficult to understand someone speaking if a vacuum cleaner is running. When we do miss something we wanted to hear, the normal response is to ask the person to repeat what they said or to ask them to quit trying to discuss the meaning of life while sweeping the carpet.

For those who develop hearing loss, the perception of background noise can be very different. As a person's hearing worsens, they hear less and less of the noises that everyone else put up with on a daily basis. They may not hear their own footsteps or the furnace running or road and wind noise when in a car. One by one, they no longer hear many of the sounds that surround them and may forget how they ignored or "tuned out" these sounds. Conversely, they continue to hear the radio and television well because they can turn it up

46

louder. Their family and friends intentionally or unintentionally begin to speak louder so they are heard and understood. The person's world becomes fairly quiet with the exception of family and friends who speak louder and electronic devices with increased volume. Over time, the perception develops that background noise is abnormal, their family and friends speak at a normal level and everyone else mumbles.

A rude awakening is often in store for those hearing impaired persons who have their hearing improved or restored through surgery or hearing aids. All of a sudden they hear not just those things they wanted, but the surrounding sounds also. In addition to hearing what they wanted, they hear the furnace, the dishwasher and their stomach growling. And for some reason, their family and friends are now yelling at them.

The people who have their hearing improved through surgery are the ones who adapt most quickly to again living in a world of sound. Whether they like their new hearing level or not, they are thrown twenty-four hours a day into a noisy world. They get used to it. For those who begin wearing hearing aids to improve their hearing, the rate at which they get used to the surrounding sounds is related to how much they wear the hearing aids. The improved hearing levels (including the background noise) will seem more natural to the person who wears their hearing aids through most of their waking hours. It is what they become used to. On the other hand, those who only wear their hearing aids occasionally will be most used to hearing without them. Their use will remain foreign or unnatural, background noise with the aids will remain annoying, and family and friends will seem to be yelling.

Regardless of what we are told by some of the advertisements on television, it is actually unrealistic to expect someone to design a device that will eliminate all forms of background noise. Two people would be unlikely to agree on what sounds they considered background noise. Even for one person, the definition of background noise would likely change from one situation to another. Especially difficult would be defining background noise in a group of people. Aside from the person you want to hear, everyone else would be background noise. Which person would you choose to hear?

There are, however, devices to help people overcome noise in a variety of specific situations. Some of these make it easier to hear the television, the teacher in a classroom or the actors on a stage. Most of these work by placing a microphone very close to what a person is trying to hear, relative to the things they do not want to hear. These devices do not actually filter out unwanted sounds. Instead, they effectively get a person closer to what they want to hear.

Rather than trying to eliminate background noise from a hearing impaired person's world, the goal should be to bring them back into the world of sound the rest of us experience.

Noise Pollution

The other noise bugaboo is noise pollution. Although annoying, noise is not something that would generally be thought of as a pollutant by most people. It does not taste bad, leave soot on our houses or leave dead fish floating around. Further, the environmental protection agency is not known for going out of the way to post signs about it. Despite this, noise pollution affects many people.

There are many sounds that could be considered pollution. Some would classify rap or rock music as noise pollution. Others might feel opera fits into this category. There would certainly be pretty good agreement about disco. Excluding arguments about music, the sounds that need to be classified as noise pollution are those that detract from the natural environment and are distracting or offensive to most people. Examples of these sounds might include noise from traffic, airplanes, railroads, industry, lawn mowers, household appliances and power tools. Aside from their intended function, the sound from each can serve to make life less pleasant or more difficult for someone else. It is hard to learn in school if a jack hammer is pounding away outside. Getting over a headache will be difficult for a person living next to a blast zone. Sleeping is likely to be less restful for a person who hears police and fire sirens all night.

Many of the sounds in a modern industrial society are necessary and we have to live with them. Others can be eliminated or limited in some way to make them less bothersome. Cities often develop noise ordinances prohibiting sounds above a certain level or loud sounds too late at night. Dishwasher, garbage disposal and other appliance manufacturers strive to make their premium appliances as quiet as possible (not necessarily the cheaper ones). Companies realize that quiet can be a selling point, and they take advantage of it when convenient. When it is not convenient, the noise prevails.

As individuals, we are limited in how much we can control noise pollution. We can insulate the walls of our houses to block some outside sounds and buy quieter appliances to keep the inside sounds soft. However, once outside, we are often out of luck. If there are local noise ordinances, a person could report every neighbor, passerby or industry that makes too much noise. However, this can be as aggravating as the noise. Often there are no local noise ordinances and the point is moot.

One of the best ways to deal with noise pollution is to work out a deal with the people making the noise. If the neighbor's rock band keeps you and your children awake when they are practicing, ask if they could practice earlier when the kids are awake. If another neighbor cuts their yard at 6:00 a.m. every Saturday morning, you might express concern for their health. You could tell them that their blood pressure is likely to be much higher first thing in the morning and that it would be safer for them to cut the yard later in the day. You may not have to explain that the greatest danger to their health is really from you.

Often the noise pollution to which we are exposed is here to stay regardless of what we think about it. Our choice may be to live with it or move away. If a freeway is built next to your house, it is unlikely you will be able to get all of the cars and trucks to drive by quietly. Similarly, it would not be too bright to buy a house at the end of an airport runway and then complain about the noise. If the noise is too much and you can't change it, the best solution may be to deal with it by moving away and moving on.

Chapter Three: Hearing Through The Years

Infants

The majority of children are born healthy and hearing well. In most cases the issue of hearing is never even questioned by new parents. After surviving the delivery, tests, hospital stay and insurance dealings, if there were time to worry about something, it would likely not be hearing.

After all, why would we be concerned with what an infant hears? It's not like we're worried about their getting a job at this age. It is also not a safety issue. There is very little probability that an infant will drive a cement mixer over someone because they couldn't hear the warnings of others. Many of the quality of life issues such as not being able to hear well enough to disco or to fully enjoy the sound track from a Kung-fu movie also don't apply to infants. What does it matter if a child goes a few years before anyone suspects or discovers their hearing loss?

The major concern about infants with hearing loss is the possibility of delayed or poor language development. Obviously, if kids can't hear words, they will be less likely to say them. Each day a childhood hearing loss goes undiscovered represents more time that will be wasted and more effort that will be required to try to catch up. Early childhood is a critical time for language development. It is much easier to learn language during early childhood. Anyone who has tried to learn a second language as an adult can attest to this. Because of this critical period for language development, children whose hearing loss was discovered later generally have more difficulty learning language than if the loss had been discovered earlier. The longer the hearing loss goes undiscovered, the less likely it will be for a child's language to develop to its full potential. Finally, limited language skills usually mean limited reading skills and poor academic achievement.

Considering that most kids hear well and do not have a hearing loss, who should be tested? Ideally, every child would have their hearing checked at birth. In this way, no children with congenital hearing loss would be missed. There are many advocates for testing the hearing of all children shortly following birth (universal hearing screening). However, ours is not an ideal world and in the midst of many other worthwhile programs such as childhood immunizations, head start, and providing prenatal care to expectant mothers, funding for universal hearing screening is not always seen as a major priority.

Years ago, few infants were tested. Hearing was only checked for the children who didn't learn to talk. Smaller hearing losses were discovered during school hearing screenings. More recently, infants are referred for a hearing test on the basis of a high risk register. This register is a list of things that have been shown to be associated with hearing loss. Some of the things that would put a child at a greater than average risk for hearing loss would include a family history of nerve hearing loss, meningitis, the need for oxygen at birth, prenatal illness of the mother (German measles, chicken pox, etc.) and low birth weight. A high risk register would list these and a number of other possible indicators for hearing loss. If a risk factor appears in the child's history, then a hearing test is performed. If there does not appear to be any risk factors for hearing loss, then a hearing test is not performed. Parental suspicion of a hearing loss or the child not seeming to respond appropriately to sound would also indicate the need for a test.

Now that we have discussed which infants are tested, it is time to explain how they are tested. At first it might appear that it would be very difficult to determine what infants can hear. They most certainly are not going to tell us. We can watch them to see what sounds they consistently respond to, but infants usually only respond to very loud sounds. They may startle, blink their eyes, wrinkle their face, drool or emit other bodily fluids in response to these loud sounds, but not for the soft ones. This might let us rule out total deafness, but it is of limited value in determining whether they can hear normally.

The primary method of testing infants' hearing is with the auditory brainstem response (ABR) test. This may also be called brainstem evoked response (BER), brainstem auditory evoked response (BAER) or auditory evoked potential (AEP) testing. Regardless of what the test is called, it can measure an infant's hearing without their consciously or reflexively responding to the sound. The test is performed by taping an electrode (a small metal disk about 1/4 inch in diameter connected to a thin wire) to the forehead and behind each ear or on the earlobes. Clicking sounds are presented to the ear through an earphone and then the brain's electrical response to the sounds is recorded through the electrodes. The recording looks like a bunch of squiggly lines. However, these squiggles tend to be consistent from infant to infant and from test to test in the same infant thus making interpretation of the response relatively easy. The hearing level can be measured by presenting softer and softer clicks to find the lowest level at which the proper squiggles can be seen. The test can take as little as 20 minutes or more than an hour to perform. It is painless and reliable.

A new test that is being used to screen infants for hearing loss is called otoacoustic emissions (OAE). In this test, loud sounds are presented to the ear through an earplug earphone. If there is normal inner ear function, the ear produces a small sound of its own which is then measured back through the same earplug earphone. This returned sound is also seen as a set of characteristic squiggles (though different from the ABR / BER / BAER / AEP squiggles). If the proper squiggles can be seen, then the hearing is considered to be normal. If the proper squiggles are not seen, then a possible hearing loss is indicated. Otoacoustic emissions are used as a pass / fail test. It is not used to measure the amount of hearing loss. As OAE testing proves itself reliable, it is becoming the primary hearing screening test for infants. Because OAE testing is faster (about 5 minutes) and easier than ABR testing, it is making universal hearing screening practical and affordable, in addition to desirable.

Children

As previously noted, hearing loss is not a problem that we would associate with childhood. Mumps, measles, and chicken pox are the illnesses that quickly come to mind for children. Focusing strictly on the ears, we might think of ear infections or ears stuffed full of mashed potatoes, but most likely not hearing loss. We do not expect or want to accept the idea of a child that does not hear well. We might expect this for an eighty-year-old man who spent his early working years as a tank commander and his later years as a jack hammer operator. Who wouldn't? But children rarely spend much time in tanks, around jack hammers or other noises identified as causing hearing loss.

Whether we like it or not, some children start out their young lives with hearing loss. Although less than one percent of children are born with hearing loss, these are often the most profound and least medically correctable cases. Many of these losses are due to a genetic malformation causing the hearing nerves to develop improperly. Others are caused by infection or disease producing the same result. If these children are not tested at birth as part of a hearing screening program, their hearing losses often go unnoticed until their speech fails to develop. Treatment for these nerve hearing losses consists of hearing aids to make sound loud enough for the child to hear. Treatment also consists of speech therapy to correct speech and language delays. Additionally, special educational plans are designed to prevent or minimize educational delays. In the few cases where the loss is too advanced for hearing aids, a cochlear implant (discussed later) is another option to improve the hearing.

Fortunately, the majority of hearing losses seen in children are much milder and generally correctable. The usual culprit is ear infections. The middle ear fills up with fluid not letting the sound get through to the hearing nerves. The fluid may not actually be infected, but either way, it can lower the hearing. If there is only a little bit of thin fluid, there may be little hearing loss. If there is a lot of fluid or the fluid is thick like glue, there may be a significant hearing loss. The hearing can fluctuate from day to day or from week to week between these two extremes. Antibiotics are the first treatment used to cure the infection and eliminate the fluid. In cases where the infection or fluid remains after multiple antibiotics or where there are repeated ear infections, it may be necessary for a doctor to put a nick in the eardrum, drain the fluid and insert a ventilation tube in the drum to prevent the fluid from reoccurring. Once the fluid is gone and the eardrum and ear bones can move properly, the hearing returns to normal. If there has been a long history of repeated ear infections, speech and language therapy is sometimes needed to correct delays caused by the hearing loss.

Regardless of the cause or degree, hearing loss in children is a major concern. Very young children need to learn speech and language. Any period where they cannot hear properly is like "time out." Other kids just pass them by. Even if it is possible to correct the child's hearing later, they may have more difficulty understanding their lessons in school due to the corresponding language delays. Hearing loss during the school years can affect more than speech development. It can impact a child's entire life. If a child is not hearing well enough to learn the fundamentals of reading, writing, arithmetic, etc., they are less likely to do well in the higher grades or in college. With a limited education, their employment options also become limited. When care is taken to identify children with a hearing loss early, improve the hearing as much as possible, correct or minimize the associated speech, language and educational delays, then there is the potential for a much brighter future.

For the few children whose hearing cannot be medically corrected and require hearing aids, there is sometimes concern that they will be viewed as disabled or handicapped. However, needing hearing aids should not be seen as a handicap. Not hearing is the handicap. Hearing aids should be accepted like eye glasses. If hearing aids allow a child to develop good speech and language skills as well as allowing them to excel at school, then there is no effective disability. The possibility does exist that a child will view him or herself as handicapped or that others will view them as handicapped for wearing hearing aids. However, despite looking less handicapped without hearing aids, they run the risk of instead appearing mentally or developmentally disabled because they respond inappropriately to what is said. After years spent in school not hearing the things they should have, and consequently not having learned them, effectively they would be disabled.

Adults

After disheartening everyone with the fact that infants and children can have hearing loss, some might be surprised to hear that adulthood (old age excluded) is normally the golden age of hearing. By this time we are usually past the ear infections of childhood and any associated hearing loss. We are also past the curiosity of childhood that might lead us to insert items of interest (peanuts, play-doh, crayons etc.) into our ears for lack of anything better to do. Accidents, stupidity, disease and years of noise may eventually take their toll on a person's hearing, but this is not often a daily concern of most adults. For the majority, hearing during adulthood is like having the sun rise in the morning or set at night. Hearing well is just the way things are and it does not do a whole lot of good to worry about it too much.

Listening as an adult is much easier than listening as a child. Less of what is heard is new. We have already learned language, attended school and had a number of years to have been there and done that. This being the case, we are more likely to be aware if something is misheard or did not sound right. Adults also have a larger range of knowledge and experience from which to fill in the few things that might have been missed. Finally, adults have greater freedom to change or avoid the few situations where they may not hear well.

With adulthood also comes greater focus. We have a better understanding of what we want to listen to and how to pay attention to it. A singer listens to make sure their voice is on pitch. A machinist listens to make sure their equipment is operating properly. Anyone who has taken a child hunting or bird watching will quickly notice how much difficulty they have hearing and distinguishing the different animal and environmental sounds. Children do not yet know which sounds are important or how to focus on them. All of these things are a matter of learning. But, having been learned, they make it possible to hear better.

Adulthood is not necessarily the time in our lives when we hear the best. However, it is often the time when we can make the best use of our hearing or when our hearing is least likely to let us down. The combination of learning, experience and situational factors during adulthood all combine with our still pretty good hearing to effectively give us super hearing. These things let us reach beyond what we already hear well, to make out what we might otherwise almost hear. Disease, trauma, accidents or noise may eventually take away some of the hearing on which this is built. But until then, every day can be a sunny day in ear land.

Baby Boomers

The baby boom generation has always been considered as a special group. Right from the start, they began shaping their world. When they were born, the size and number of maternity wards had to be dramatically increased so they would all fit. The nation became obsessed with finding better and more scientific methods of child care. They hoped these hoards would grow up to be happy, well adjusted, hardworking adults rather than malcontent robbers, rapists and murderers. The result landed somewhere between these two extremes. They got hippies and rock and roll. The shear quantity of baby boomers forced changes in medicine, schools, colleges, the workplace and society in general. As they are getting older, we see greater and greater concern about social security, retirement, health care that is available and responsive to the needs of seniors, and a whole variety of other age related issues. We are even starting to see television commercials geared toward and starring someone other than teenagers. The media continues to hold up a teenage image as the goal everyone should strive for, but more and more, the baby boomers are telling the media to get real. Their teen years are gone and no amount of diet or exercise is going to get them back into their purple and orange plaid polyester elephant bells (or the current equivalent thereof).

Of concern here are possible factors that might put aging baby boomers at greater risk for hearing loss than previous generations. Baby boomers are the first generation to spend their entire lives exposed to electrically amplified music. It may only be rock and roll, but it is loud. Whether at the front row of a rock concert, in a basement club, in the car or at home under headphones, the music can be loud enough to gradually damage the hearing nerves. During a lifetime of this, the damage accumulates.

Another factor putting aging baby boomers at greater risk of eventually developing hearing loss is a longer life span during which this can happen. It is not just more years of rock and roll. It is more years for numerous diseases, noise and general wear and tear to take their toll on the ears. If they had lived long enough, earlier generations might have had these same problems. However, they didn't, so age related hearing loss was not a major concern until recently.

As the number of older baby boomers grows, so will the emphasis on age related problems. The great numbers and political clout of the baby boomers almost guarantee it. There will likely also be greater demand for better or more complete insurance coverage for the diagnosis and treatment of hearing problems, as well as for hearing aids if the loss cannot be medically or surgically corrected. While uncommon now, obtaining complete coverage for something like hearing aids would be a minor change compared to all of the other ways the baby boomers have changed society.

The Later Years

Although hearing may gradually worsen with age, aging in and of itself does not cause hearing loss. The ears are not programmed to self-destruct at any particular time. Hearing losses attributed to age are often a side effect of health problems associated with aging, or years of wear and tear on the body in general or on the ears specifically. People who have had less wear and tear on their ears (less noise exposure, fewer medications that might damage hearing etc.) often have good hearing even into old age. The few people in remote non-industrial societies who manage to survive to become old, usually have much better hearing than their counterparts from industrialized societies. They have not worn their ears out with the sounds and substances of modern life.

One functional change related to aging is the speed at which our brain processes what we hear. Children and very young adults process sound very quickly. They understand what is said the instant they hear it. Starting around our thirties, it begins to take a little longer for our brains to process the sounds provided by our ears. It takes longer for us to understand what is said: to "get" it. In most listening situations this is not much of a problem. However, if a person is listening to someone talking fast or if there are a lot of things going on at the same time, it becomes more and more difficult to keep up. We may understand the beginning of what was said, but miss the end because we were figuring out the beginning. This gradual reduction in processing speed is a natural process. It cannot be classified as a hearing loss, but at times may produce a similar result. It can make it tougher to understand what was said. Fortunately, simple changes such as asking people to speak a little slower and reducing competing noise are successful in making up for it.

There are a number of health problems sometimes acquired during the aging process that may eventually result in hearing loss (kidney problems, high blood pressure, circulatory problems, etc.). In other cases, health problems may prohibit medical or surgical procedures that might otherwise be used to improve hearing. Age simply allows more time for these other things to cause a hearing problem or prevent the problem from being corrected. However, in most cases, a hearing loss that could have been medically or surgically treated for a younger adult can also be treated for an older adult.

Since hearing may decline very gradually with age, many people are unaware that they no longer hear well. They may seem to hear as well today as they did the day before, and they do not seem to hear any worse than their friends the same age. Further, their listening demands usually lessen with age making it less likely for a hearing loss to be noticed. Family members get used to talking a little louder to make sure they are heard and understood. Their peers are likely to talk a little louder because they cannot hear well either. But eventually, they begin to notice that others are hearing things that they do not. These individuals may wish to pursue hearing aids to replace some of the sound that nature has taken away.

Chapter Four: The Professionals

Ear Doctors

Just as there are foot doctors for feet and heart doctors for hearts, there are ear doctors for ears. All they do, all day long, are ears. There are also doctors that specialize in several areas, one of which is ears. All of these physicians are real doctors with medical and surgical training who graduated from accredited medical or osteopathic schools. They have passed written and oral board examinations as well as meeting all of the educational and legal requirements of the states in which they practice. These were kids who did well in school.

The best known of the ear doctors are the ear, nose and throat (ENT) doctors. As the name implies, they treat nose and throat problems in addition to ear problems. They are also known as otolaryngologists. A less commonly known ear doctor is an otologist. They focus strictly on the ears. Even more specialized are neurotologists. These physicians also focus strictly on the ears but have additional training.

Ear doctors are specialists in diagnosing or ruling out ear diseases. These include, but are not limited to, those that cause hearing loss. In order to make a proper diagnosis the physician takes a detailed history, performs a physical examination and orders tests that will aid in the diagnosis. Most ear doctors have an audiologist on staff so the needed tests can be performed on the initial visit. Experienced ear doctors will usually need very little time to make a diagnosis once all the information is available. When a diagnosis is reached, the doctor will explain what can or cannot be done. This is sometimes the most time consuming part of the visit since it is often necessary to educate the patient about their particular ear disease before they can make an informed decision about any treatment options.

Medications or treatment programs can be prescribed by ear doctors to treat or manage many different ear diseases. When the damage to the ear is unaffected or not treatable by medication, surgery may be possible to correct the problem. A torn or punctured eardrum can be patched, broken or eroded ear bones can be replaced, and fluid or infection in the middle ear can be drained to allow the ear to work properly. If there is severe damage to the inner ear, the remaining hearing nerves can be electrically stimulated to restore hearing through the use of a cochlear implant. These and other surgical procedures to repair structures, eliminate disease and to improve or preserve hearing are performed by ear doctors. If it is possible to fix an ear, these are the people who do it.

Audiologists

Regardless of what the name implies, audiologists do not sell stereo equipment. Audiologists are trained to perform, interpret and counsel people regarding just about every hearing and ear related test with the exception of imaging studies (MRIs and X-rays). Audiologists are also university trained in the prescription, fitting and evaluation of hearing aids and assistive listening devices. Although audiologists are licensed to practice independently, they often work for or with ear doctors for a number of practical considerations. The two professions can work very well as a team. Audiologists perform the tests ear doctors need to make a diagnosis. Once a diagnosis is reached, the ear doctor can work with the people who can be helped medically or surgically and the audiologist can work with the people who must compensate for their hearing loss with hearing aids, assistive listening devices or individualized listening strategies.

The majority of audiologists have a Master's degree in audiology. This is the clinical degree in the field. There are Ph.D. audiologists, but most of these teach audiology and perform research in universities rather than practicing clinically. Training as an audiologist includes course work in hearing, speech, language, anatomy and physiology of the ears, the acoustics of sound, statistics, research methods and electronics, in addition to all of the courses universities routinely require for a balanced education. Also required before a degree is awarded are hundreds of supervised clinical hours with patients. National testing is performed by an independent organization to insure the competency of audiologists entering practice. Following graduation, a beginning audiologist must work for a year under the supervision of an experienced audiologist before they can practice independently. Audiology training is unique and should not be confused with medical school. It is a separate career path.

Audiologists come in many shapes, sizes and use various titles. Years ago, the majority of audiologists were male. With greater numbers of women entering the work force and excelling in technical and professional fields, a person is more likely to have a female audiologist today. The majority of these professionals are known as clinical audiologists. They work directly with people in clinical settings. However, there are different designations based on the audiologist's individual training or on their experience with a particular patient population. Audiologists working in the schools are known as educational audiologists. Those working primarily with children are known as pediatric audiologists. Industrial audiologists monitor hearing and noise levels in industry. Research audiologists monitor the effectiveness of current procedures as well as develop and evaluate new ear and hearing related procedures. There are other areas of specialization in this field, but you get the idea.

Hearing Aid Dealers

Years ago, the only people who sold hearing aids were hearing aid dealers. The hearing aids were big, ugly and considered as more of a gadget than a medical device. The few audiologists practicing at the time did not sell hearing aids due to a perceived conflict of interest with their testing and counseling roles. In this environment, hearing aid dealers acquired their clients by default. No one else wanted to sell hearing aids. They saw potential benefit for their clients and profits for themselves. It was an exciting new field and they were taking a hand in creating and shaping it. In some ways, they were not dissimilar to many of the early computer "nerds". They did not have a formal education in what they were doing, but the field was new enough that this did not put them at a significant disadvantage. They could help people and earn a good living at the same time.

Hearing aid dealers today will often have apprenticed themselves for a period with an experienced hearing aid dealer to learn their trade. They might also have completed some form of hearing aid course or seminar offered by a university or hearing aid manufacturer. States require hearing aid dealers to pass a test before they are licensed to sell hearing aids. They are not, however, usually required to have formal medical or audiological training from an accredited university. This lack of formal education often puts them at a disadvantage to university trained audiologists who now sell hearing aids in addition to their other audiologic duties. The wider range of services provided by audiologists usually results in their being more closely allied with general practitioners and ear doctors than are hearing aid dealers. Many of the hearing aid referrals that used to go to hearing aid dealers, now go to audiologists. Seeing the handwriting on the wall, many of the people who would have become hearing aid dealers if they were starting their careers years ago, today make use of the university training available and become audiologists instead.

Hearing instrument specialist (HIS) is the preferred and politically correct title for a hearing aid dealer today. A hearing instrument specialist is not necessarily more or less a specialist in hearing aids than a hearing aid dealer. The title simply sounds more impressive which explains this preference in terminology. An even more impressive, but more difficult title is auditory prosthologist. The name makes a lot of sense if we consider a hearing aid as a prosthesis. However, barring someone writing a really catchy jingle, the term auditory prosthologist seems unlikely to catch on. For simplicity, anyone selling hearing aids (hearing aid dealer, audiologist, physician, etc.) will be referred to as a hearing aid fitter for the remainder of the book.

All of the terminology put aside, hearing aid dealers sell hearing aids. They are not usually physicians, audiologists or medically trained professionals. They are salespeople specializing in hearing aids. Given years of experience, they can be very good at providing the best hearing aid fitting possible. The skill level of a beginning hearing aid dealer may be less certain.

Speech And Language Pathologists

It would be inappropriate to write a book about hearing and hearing loss without also explaining the role of speech and language pathologists. Like audiologists, they have earned at least a master's degree from an accredited university, passed a national standards test and practiced a year under the direct supervision of someone more experienced. Unlike audiologists, the majority of their training is in speech and language development and pathology, rather than hearing. They are expert in determining whether speech and language are developing at a normal rate or in some abnormal way. They are also expert in creating and implementing plans to correct or treat these abnormalities. They may occasionally perform hearing screenings, but this is not their primary role.

Although speech and language pathologists do not diagnose or treat hearing loss, they are important to many of the hearing impaired because they are the ones who diagnose and treat some of the results of hearing loss. These results

68

might include delayed, abnormal or nonexistent speech and language development or the gradual degradation of speech following the onset of a severe or profound hearing loss. They clean up some of the mess a hearing loss may create.

Children with hearing loss are less likely to develop speech and language at a normal rate or in a normal manner. They are not very likely to learn speech if they cannot hear it well or if they cannot hear it at all. Equally confusing can be all of the things that they hear, but hear incorrectly. It is the job of the speech language pathologist to help these children learn the speech and language that they have not learned, unlearn what they have heard wrong and to develop plans to keep them progressing normally despite their hearing loss.

Less recognized is what can happen to a person's speech after developing a large hearing loss. Even if a person has had normal speech and hearing for years, the quality, clarity, or loudness of a person's speech can change drastically following the onset of a severe hearing loss. If the hearing loss becomes large enough, the person can no longer hear and monitor what they are saying. Their voice can become loud, monotone or they may slur their words together. This voice quality is sometimes referred to as "deaf speech." The speech and language pathologist has to identify the specific ways these people are slaughtering their speech and help them find ways to correct it.

Speech and language pathologists who work with the hearing impaired often do so as part of a team that also includes an ear doctor and audiologist. The speech pathologist's role is normally very small for people having mild hearing losses. However, their role greatly increases for people who have larger hearing losses. They help hearing impaired children learn to talk, and they help hearing impaired adults keep talking. If not technically one of the "ear people," speech and language pathologists definitely belong among them.

Others

Ear doctors, audiologists and hearing aid fitters are not the only people who do ear stuff. There are others. First and foremost are primary care doctors. While their main concern is the overall health of the individual, they are often the first to hear reports of hearing difficulties or to see signs of infection or disease. Obviously the majority of their training is not in treating ear problems. However, they can treat simple ear problems or indicate the appropriate specialist to see for problems that are beyond their practice.

Pediatricians are another group of specialists that see many ear problems. In fact, ear infections are one of the most common problems they see. Fortunately, the majority of these infections clear up with antibiotics. During the course of the overall examination, pediatricians also have to be aware of anything that might indicate a possible hearing loss (family history, certain complications before or at birth, delayed speech or language development, etc.). Some pediatricians will screen the hearing of the children they see, but the majority refer their patients to an ear doctor or audiologist if there is the suspicion of a potential hearing loss.

Another group involved in ear evaluations are audiometric technicians. These are individuals who are usually trained by an ear doctor to perform hearing, balance or other ear related tests. They only work under the direction of a physician and are not permitted to perform these services without supervision (however, laws do vary somewhat from state to state). Although they may perform a variety of tests, technicians do not interpret the results. This is done by an ear doctor. Audiometric technicians used to be fairly common, but have largely been replaced by audiologists who can perform and interpret tests without supervision. The university and clinical training required to become an audiologist also insures a higher level of competence for the patient that is not always guaranteed in the case of a technician.

School systems also test hearing. In order to teach kids, it is very important to first make sure the children can hear the person trying to teach them. Schools routinely screen the hearing of children before they enter kindergarten. They may also check them every few years or if there is a suspected problem. The employees the schools use for these tests vary widely. Some schools have audiologists for these purposes, but many do not. Due to funding constraints, schools will often use whomever they have at hand. They may use school nurses, speech pathologists, teachers, teacher aides or even parent volunteers. Some are trained to screen hearing, some are not. While using minimally trained or untrained individuals to perform hearing screenings may not be optimal, it is better than nothing. At least some of the children with hearing loss are detected and pointed in the right direction for a full evaluation.

The main point here is that ear doctors, audiologists and hearing aid dealers are not the only ones who see people with ear or hearing problems. If a person has ear disease or hearing loss, they will usually end up seeing an ear doctor, audiologist or possibly a hearing aid fitter, but it is not unusual for them to first see others that direct them along the way.

Experience Matters

As a society, we do not always show a great deal of reverence or respect for age and experience. Rather than putting the most experienced person in charge, we have mandatory retirement. Rather than companies striving to fill their work forces with experienced people, we have had to pass laws to keep many of these companies from eliminating their older workers to reduce costs. Instead of equating age with wisdom and experience, our society equates age with inflexibility and obsolescence. Just as in the advertisements for new products, we also want professionals who will do things the new and improved way. Knowledge, experience and a proven track record may be overshadowed by a quest for something new.

Regardless of society's views, experience does matter. There is a big difference between having once read about a disease in a book and having correctly identified it a thousand times. There is a big difference between having read about or watched a surgical procedure and having successfully performed it many times. Experience is especially important when a disease appears to be something else or when a surgical procedure does not go as planned. An experienced doctor will have been in this position before and will know from experience what worked and what did not. This may be virgin territory for the less experienced. Doctors specialize for this very reason. They can become expert by focusing on one or a limited number of diseases or procedures. In fact, there is a learning curve for some surgical procedures that extends well beyond school. Successful surgical results are more likely to be obtained once a doctor has performed a specific procedure more than a certain number of times. For those experienced at a particular procedure, it may also be necessary to perform a certain number each year for skill maintenance. There is a reason some people with difficult or exotic medical problems will travel halfway around the world to see a particular specialist. Experience can make a difference in the outcome.

Clearly, experience is an important consideration when choosing an ear doctor. It is also an important consideration if choosing an audiologist, hearing aid dealer or other ear professional. Ear related tests may be more accurate when performed by someone more experienced. Hearing aids fit by an experienced person may be more comfortable and outperform those fit by a less experienced person (due to the most appropriate hearing aid style or circuitry having been selected for the person's individual hearing loss and lifestyle).

For those procedures (hearing screenings, hearing aid fitting, fitting earplugs, wax removal, etc.) that may be performed by professionals having differing levels or areas of training, years of education for one professional may need to be weighed against years of experience for another. We may choose to be fitted by a hearing aid dealer having little formal training but years of experience successfully fitting patients, instead of by a beginning audiologist with a college degree, but no track record. Similarly, many of the people who perform hearing screenings have become good at this through years of experience rather than through formal education. We may choose to make use of one of these individuals because of their past performance, rather than someone university trained, but inexperienced.

Education is very important, but experience matters also. We would all be best served by the most educated and experienced professionals available, but we often have to choose between degrees of these two. Society may favor the trendy and new, but this does not mean that we would be best served by people untrained, inexperienced or unproven. Experience matters.

White Coats

Medical people wear white coats. We are all taught this from earliest childhood and it has become somewhat expected for ear people also. While wearing a white coat does not mean a person graduated from medical school, we often react as if it did. Television goes out of its way to play on and foster this view. Imagine a medical show where the doctors did not wear their traditional doctor coats. We might be less likely to find them interesting and more likely to consider their lines less dramatic if not at times really stupid. Similarly, we would be unlikely to pay much credence to television sales people pitching headache, diarrhea or hemorrhoid relievers if they were not wearing white coats.

When people are bleeding, oozing or otherwise leaking something, lab coats offer some small degree of protection for the professionals wearing them. Those working in emergency rooms or urgent care centers all wear lab coats or some other form of protective clothing. The clothing protects them and can be changed if contaminated. Other hospital staff may also wear special clothing for the same purposes. Aside from physicians and nurses, most ear people (audiologists, hearing aid dealers, technicians etc.) are less likely to need special dress for ear battle. They may occasionally want to put on a lab coat or gloves if performing wax removals or when taking an earmold impression for a hearing aid, but this is not a necessity for the majority of work they do.

Although some medical professionals need to wear white coats, there are others who wear them simply to look like doctors or give the impression that they are doctors. This doesn't just happen on television. Some people play doctor in real life. When this does happen, we need to keep in mind that white coats in and of themselves mean nothing. Competence is based on training and experience, not the outfit worn. Rather than looking at their white coat, look for degrees on their office walls and ask them how long they have been practicing.

Insurance And Your Ears

The majority of us have some form of medical insurance. However, the amount or type of coverage varies greatly from person to person and from insurance plan to insurance plan. Almost all plans cover major medical problems like heart attack or stroke. Insurance coverage for conditions that are not life threatening are less certain. Ear and hearing problems are usually grouped with these not life threatening problems. Occasionally, the diagnosis or treatment of these problems is defined as medically unnecessary and insurance coverage is denied. Sometimes the methods used to determine coverage are understandable and well thought out, other times not.

The very first thing anyone suspecting an ear or hearing problem should do is call their insurance company. Find out whether your plan includes coverage for ear or hearing problems. If insurance coverage is provided, ask if there is any rule as to which professional(s) may be seen, or if a referral is needed in order to obtain insurance reimbursement for seeing a specialist. Some plans may require the policy holder to see their primary care doctor first. It is always a good idea to get the name of the person at the insurance company you are talking with in case there is any later dispute or misunderstanding about coverage.

Under some insurance plans it is much easier for the policy holder to determine who they may see for an ear problem, than what may or may not be covered by their policy. The majority of medical plans will cover an examination by an ear doctor. However, some do not cover hearing related tests. This kind of coverage lets the ear doctor say with certainty that the ears look like ears, but often leaves them no closer to making a diagnosis because the needed tests are not covered. Other insurance plans will cover the ear examination and tests, unless they are performed to select a hearing aid. Conversely, there are insurance plans that will pay for the physical examination and tests only if they are performed to select a hearing aid. However, more often than not, coverage for hearing aids is denied by insurance. Finally, everyone's favorite are the plans that determine reimbursement on the basis of the ear examination and test results. The insurance companies reimburse based on the diagnosis, which of course, is impossible for the patient or physician to know prior to the examination and tests.

Pretty obviously, insurance companies are not ear people. They may not even have an ear specialist reviewing the claims. However, by holding the purse strings, they can control which ear people are seen and influence which tests and procedures are performed. A person should trust their doctor to determine what is the best evaluation and treatment for an ear or hearing problem. But, no one should be too surprised if their insurance company disagrees.

Who Ya Gonna Call?

Most people would not have a clue who to call if they had a hearing loss or an ear problem. They could ask a friend, co-worker, grocery store clerk or personal psychic, but there would be a good chance that these others would not have a clue who to call either. Despite the high incidence of ear problems and hearing loss, we have not been educated what to do should it happen to us. We would not even know where to look for the information. If we searched out the information most readily available, it would likely be supplied in the form of a commercial with someone trying to sell us a hearing aid. The situation is not unlike trying to discern the healthiest, most thirst quenching drink by watching beer commercials.

Ideally, we would all like to be seen by, and get our information from, the best educated and most experienced ear professional possible. But which professional? Ear doctors, audiologists, hearing aid dealers, technicians and other professionals all see people with ear problems. However, they do not all do the same things. Audiologists and hearing aid dealers do not perform surgery or make medical diagnoses. Ear doctors do not generally fit hearing aids or assistive listening devices (however, they may have others that do it for them). Knowing which ear professional is needed is dependent on the nature of the ear problem. The nature of the ear problem often cannot be known without seeing an ear professional. To get away from this circular argument of which ear professional a person ultimately needs to see, a more reasonable approach is to focus on which professional it would be best to start with.

The place to start is dependent on who your insurance company will reimburse you for seeing, as well as the professionals that are available in your area. Many insurance plans require their patients to first be evaluated by their primary care physician (family doctor) before being seen by a specialist. Ear problems are no exception to this policy. The primary care doctor can treat or rule out some simple problems and if necessary, recommend a qualified specialist based on what they see. People can start with someone they know and trust (their primary care doctor) and, if a referral is needed, have greater confidence that they are seeing the appropriate specialist and that they are qualified. There is no need to throw darts at the medical pages of the phone book. Even if not required by insurance, seeing a primary care doctor can be a practical place to start and may be the only place to start in small towns or rural areas that are not large enough to support an ear specialist. For those with good insurance, this route usually leads to the best professionals available with a minimum amount of cost to the patient.

For those without insurance or with insurance that doesn't cover ear evaluations (a few do not), the most cost effective route for patients may be different. Some people will start at a free hearing screening offered at a church, community center or by a hearing aid dealer (hearing aid dealers love to do free hearing screenings because it can generate hearing aid sales). If the person fails the screening, only then do they consider proceeding to a medical specialist (most often the specialist recommended by the person performing the hearing screening). Others will start with a local ear professional based on the recommendation of someone they trust or because of an advertisement. Some of these people will start with a full audiologic evaluation (performed by an audiologist). This will show the degree, severity, and location of the hearing loss. It will also give an indication of the cause, as well as whether it might be correctable. This kind of evaluation can rule out hearing loss, show if hearing aids would be helpful and indicate when a medical referral should be pursued. Audiologists do charge for their services, but not nearly as much as ear doctors.

People with a previously diagnosed ear problem can often go directly to the specialist they need for follow-up (insurance permitting). Those having had medication or surgery to restore or preserve hearing will follow-up with their ear doctor. If yearly hearing tests are needed to monitor hearing levels, people can go directly to an audiologist. If a person needs to repair or replace worn out hearing aids, they can go directly to an audiologist or hearing aid dealer. People do not necessarily have to start over each time by seeing all of the medical professionals they saw the first time around. They can go directly to the person they need to see.

In summary, there are a couple of key steps in deciding which professional to see for an ear problem. The first is to check your insurance to determine whether ear examinations are covered, and if so, whether there are any specific steps required for coverage. Those knowing an ear doctor, audiologist or experienced hearing aid dealer in their area, could start with one of these professionals (provided their insurance does not specify something different). If you do not know any ear professionals (most people do not), a good starting place is your primary care doctor. They can rule out or treat simple problems and recommend a qualified ear specialist if needed. This eliminates the need for people to try to determine which ear professional is the best trained or most competent. It is certainly better than randomly picking a name out of a phone book or choosing an ear person simply because they advertise the most.

Chapter Five: Diseases And Treatment

Diagnosis Normal

The most hoped for and most common diagnosis is normal ears and hearing. Many people see ear or hearing specialists in the hope of ruling out a suspected or feared problem. There may be a family history of a particular disease, years of noise exposure, some kind of trauma or other factor that increases their risk of an ear or hearing problem. The goal in getting an examination is to be sure that these things have not taken any toll. The majority who find this to be the case, return home reassured that they are OK and all is right in their world.

In some cases, the expected diagnosis is normal hearing. This is true when large numbers of people are being screened to rule out a problem. These screenings might be for children entering school, recruits entering the service or employees entering a new job. The screenings make sure the majority hear well and identify the few who will need a more extensive evaluation.

For some, a diagnosis of normal ears and hearing may not be viewed as good news. A parent may be more likely to hope for a diagnosis of hearing loss (preferably a correctable one) as the cause of their child's speech and language delays, than for learning disabilities or mental retardation to be the cause. A hearing loss might be the preferred cause for seeming confusion in a parent, than for Alzheimer's disease to be responsible. Given certain choices, hearing loss can be the preferred situation.

For other people, a diagnosis of normal ears or hearing is no news. It is only an indicator of the need to look further. When the ear examination for a patient with ear pain is normal, then less frequent causes such as a bad tooth or problems with the jaw joint can be explored. In this case and many others, a normal ear examination serves as just the first chapter in a longer detective story.

A diagnosis of normal ears and hearing can also be a disappointment to those who truly have normal hearing but still want or need to hear better. These are often people who live or work in very demanding listening situations. A waitress in a noisy restaurant or bar may have great difficulty understanding the customers even if she has perfect hearing. A college professor may not be able to hear students questions posed from the back of the classroom. An amateur radio operator may be able to hear, but not quite discern the words of a far away radio operator. For these individuals, normal hearing is the problem. They want super hearing. They are often disappointed to find that they already have all of the hearing that nature provides. Fortunately, they can usually still benefit from lip-reading, listening strategies or assistive listening devices (described later).

Ear Infections

One of the more correctable hearing losses are those that are found to be due to an ear infection. Children are the usual targets, but infections can and do affect adults also. The general term is otitis media. This term refers to inflammation (itis) of the middle (media) ear (oto). The middle ear (the space between the eardrum and the inner ear) fills up with fluid that may or may not actually be infected. Either way, it can be uncomfortable. If the fluid becomes infected causing the eardrum to bulge outward, it is termed acute otitis media and can be very painful. If the fluid becomes thick and sticky, it may be termed glue ear or serous otitis media. Infections can also occur in the skin of the ear canal causing the ear to itch, drain or swell up. This is termed an external otitis.

The causes of otitis media are many. Children are most prone because their eustachian tubes (the little tube that supplies air to the middle ear) are not as wide as in adults and do not work as well. If the middle ears can't get air, a vacuum develops which literally sucks fluid from the surrounding tissues. Since the ear is already a nice dark warm place, adding fluid makes it almost the ideal place for germs to grow. Given time, they often do. Sore throats, tonsillitis, colds, allergies and countless other things can make the ears more prone to fluid or infection.

The primary symptoms of otitis media are hearing loss, a fullness or pressure in the ears and occasional pain or ear noise (tinnitus). Hearing loss results because the fluid that is trapped in the middle ear does not let the eardrum and ear bones move properly to transmit sound to the inner ear. Tinnitus results from the fluid or infection blocking incoming sounds that would otherwise cover up a person's head noises. The sensation of pressure or fullness is caused by the fluid actually putting pressure on or stretching the surrounding structures. This sensation can also be caused by the brain incorrectly interpreting the reduction in sound caused by the hearing loss. If the fluid becomes infected, greater pressure can build up causing pain. If the pressure created by the infection continues to build, the eardrum can burst and the ear will drain.

Given time, otitis media will sometimes resolve on its own. However, when it does not, treatment is needed to prevent the risk of fluid or infection causing long term damage to the ear. Additionally, a person is stuck not hearing well until the middle ear fluid or infection does resolve.

The primary treatment for otitis media is antibiotics. This eliminates any infection that may have developed in the middle ear and can also eliminate bacteria or infection elsewhere (in the throat or adenoids) that may have led to the ear infection in the first place. The majority of middle ear fluid and infections clear up with antibiotics. External ear infections are also treated with antibiotics (either oral or topical). They are sometimes additionally treated with a medicated earwash that gets directly at the problem.

When otitis media is not cured with antibiotics, other procedures are sometimes needed. This entails either a myringotomy or a myringotomy followed by placement in the eardrum of a ventilating tube. During a myringotomy, a small incision is made in the eardrum and the fluid or infection removed by suction. When it is found that the otitis media is due to chronic eustachian tube dysfunction, a small ventilating tube is placed in the eardrum following the myringotomy. This takes the place of the eustachian tube in supplying air to the middle ear. It also allows the eustachian tube time to mature and function better (if in a child) or simply time to get better without constantly being exposed to fluid or infection. The symptoms of pain, pressure, hearing loss and tinnitus resulting from otitis media are usually resolved immediately following the myringotomy or myringotomy and tube.

Looking ahead, ear infections may become much less common in the not too distant future. One of the new generation of vaccines being developed is likely to eliminate one of the major causes of infection: pneumococcal bacteria. Other causes will remain, but some of these may also be eradicated or at least become more treatable with the new antibiotics currently being developed.

Perforated Eardrum

An eardrum can develop a perforation (hole) in a number of ways. Infection building up behind the eardrum causing it to burst is the most common cause. A cotton swab or bobby pin pushed too far into the ear to remove wax or to scratch an itch can also tear the eardrum. Trauma of all sorts is frequently seen to stretch the eardrum beyond the breaking point. Even sparks from welding are occasionally seen to find their way into the ear canal and burn through the eardrum. A perforation can also, on occasion, result from a pressure equalization tube that has been inserted into the eardrum to control infections. The majority of the time the eardrum heals after the tube falls out or is surgically removed. But

83

sometimes, the eardrum gets used to having been held open and does not want to close after the tube comes out.

The major problems with having a hole in the eardrum are hearing loss and the ear being more prone to infection. A very small hole may have little consequence for hearing. If the hole is larger or in an inopportune place, the eardrum may not move as well and hearing loss is more likely to result. The ear also becomes more prone to infection since it is easier for moisture, dirt or assorted growies to get into the ear. If the ear does get infected, there will likely be drainage out through the eardrum perforation.

Fortunately, the majority of eardrums heal on their own within a few days of their being torn or ruptured. Many people who had a perforation years ago and still thought they had one, are amazed to find out that the eardrum fixed itself and is now just fine. However, the longer a perforation remains without healing, the less likely it will be to heal on its own. Small perforations can often be repaired by an ear doctor treating the eardrum and then placing a small paper or latex patch over the hole to serve as a template. The eardrum heals and the patch falls off or is taken off by a physician. Occasionally, the first patch will only partially do the job and the eardrum may need to be patched again before it completely heals.

When a perforation is too large to be patched or when patching is unsuccessful in closing the hole, minor surgery is possible to repair the eardrum. This form of surgery is called a tympanoplasty. During the surgery, a tissue graft is placed either on top or underneath the eardrum to repair the perforation. Following healing, these remade eardrums work very well and usually last a lifetime.

Ear Bone Damage

Ear bone (ossicular) damage refers to broken, eroded or otherwise damaged middle ear bones. Several things can do

84

this. Chronic ear infections and other middle ear pathologies are more than willing to eat their way through these tiny structures. If not totally destroyed by these afflictions, one or more of the ear bones may still need to be removed surgically to eliminate every trace of infection or disease from the ear. Trauma can also damage or destroy the little ear bones. An auto accident, being hit by a baseball, falling off the roof or taking a dive off a jet ski can all break bones. The little ear bones are no exception. There are a number of other, less frequent or traumatic ways the middle ear bones can be damaged. But, despite the odds, the damage still occurs and is every bit as real.

When the bones in the middle ear are broken or separated from one another, there is then no direct link between the eardrum and inner ear. A hearing loss results: usually a big one. The hearing nerves (hair cells) in the inner ear may be just fine, but the sound does not reach them. Not only do the little ear bones not transmit the sound, the eardrum now becomes a barrier to block sound. Without the ear bones, the eardrum is simply a wall that gets in the way of the sound.

The obvious solution to broken ear bones is to repair or replace them. In many cases, this is possible through surgery. The procedure is called an ossiculoplasty. The steps to the procedure vary depending on the severity of the damage, the cause of the hearing damage, and the preferred technique of the surgeon. But, most of the time, a connection can be reestablished that will again carry sound through the middle ear. The chance for success (a stable connection and better hearing) is better when there is only minor damage to the ear bones. However, the ear bones can often still be repaired or replaced even when there is major damage.

A hearing aid is another option for people who are reluctant or medically unable to have surgery to repair their middle ear bones. We all know that the sounds from loud cars, neighbors, stereos and barking dogs have little trouble finding their way through the walls of our homes. A hearing aid can act the same way. By making sound louder, the hearing aid overcomes the barrier created by the eardrum and missing or damaged ear bones. If the ear bones cannot be fixed, the remaining solution is to crank up the volume. Either way, the person will hear.

Cholesteatoma

Cholesteatoma is an abnormal growth of skin cells in the middle ear. The cells usually enter through a hole in the eardrum and then take on a life of their own. As the cholesteatoma develops, it harbors infection which can produce a foul smelling, draining ear. The cholesteatoma and infection can also produce a growing hearing loss as they eat away at the little ear bones and fill up the middle ear cavity. Left untreated, cholesteatoma can produce more serious consequences. This disease is most often seen in people who have had an eardrum perforation, previous ear surgery or repeated ear infections with drainage.

Surgical removal of the cholesteatoma is the required treatment for this disease. Unfortunately, since the cholesteatoma may have destroyed one or more of the little ear bones, these also may have to be removed. The surgery must be thorough because if even one small part of the cholesteatoma remains, it will grow back. Cholesteatoma is not a tumor or cancer, but it can be every bit as relentless.

To an individual, cholesteatoma may at first seem like a very minor problem. They may get a little drainage out of the ear, but still seem to hear fairly well. Even if the cholesteatoma has largely destroyed one or more of the middle ear bones, the cholesteatoma itself can transfer some of the sound through the ear. Following surgery, it is not all that uncommon for the hearing to drop because the cholesteatoma is no longer transferring the sound. The little ear bones can be replaced at the time of surgery with an artificial equivalent, but surgeons will often wait a year following the initial surgery to be sure there is no recurrence of the cholesteatoma before reconstructing the middle ear.

As far as ear diseases go, cholesteatoma is one of the nastier ones to control. Several surgeries are sometimes required before every last bit of the cholesteatoma is gone and cannot reoccur. Additionally, further surgery may be needed to replace one or more of the little ear bones in an attempt to restore the damaged hearing. Even when the cholesteatoma appears to have been completely eradicated and the hearing corrected or restored as much as possible, it is often necessary to follow these people at least yearly. The follow-ups make it possible to check for any recurrence of the disease and to provide cleaning or other needed care for an ear that has a long history of frequent infections or multiple surgeries.

Otosclerosis

Otosclerosis is a progressive ear disease in which areas of spongy bone replace healthy bone within the middle or inner ear. If this spongy growth develops on the stapes bone (the last and smallest of the ear bones) and hardens it in place, a conductive hearing loss results. This form of hearing loss is usually correctable by surgery. However, the process of otosclerotic bone replacing normal healthy bone can occur elsewhere in the ear and eventually results in a slowly progressive nerve hearing loss that is not surgically correctable. These hearing losses can be severe, but rarely does otosclerosis alone cause total deafness.

Otosclerosis is more common in women (2/3 of the cases) than in men. It usually develops during young adulthood, and in women, progresses more rapidly during pregnancy (possibly due to hormonal changes). Otosclerosis is generally considered to be hereditary. Many members of the same family may be affected, or only a few. But, most people with otosclerosis will know of at least one other relative (either close or distant) that had the disease. Otosclerosis can develop in only one ear, but most often develops in both.

The primary symptom of otosclerosis is hearing loss. The loss can be very mild or very severe if the disease has had years to progress. A person's word understanding or clarity of hearing usually remains good. It is the volume that drops off. People with otosclerosis often hear their own voice at a normal level, but the fixation of the stapes bone causes all other sounds to be blocked or very soft. This results in their retaining a normal or soft spoken voice, despite having a large hearing loss. It can also help them to retain good speech and voice quality because they can hear enough of their own voice to monitor it well. Tinnitus and unsteadiness are other symptoms sometimes reported with otosclerosis.

When the otosclerotic growth develops on the stapes bone and locks it in place, the preferred treatment is stapedectomy. This is a surgical procedure in which all or part of the stapes bone is removed and an artificial replacement inserted. Because this replacement can then move freely to transmit sound into the inner ear, the hearing improves. This procedure has been performed for more than 40 years and has a very high rate of success and a low rate of complications when performed by an experienced ear surgeon.

When the disease process results in a purely nerve hearing loss, stapedectomy is not helpful. As healthy bone is replaced by otosclerotic bone, this process can damage the nerve cells in the inner ear. An ear doctor can prescribe medications which may interrupt this process and minimize or stop further loss of hearing due to otosclerosis. If the hearing loss has progressed to a significant level and cannot be improved through surgery, hearing aids are also an option. Due to their good word understanding, people with otosclerosis usually do well if the sounds can just be made loud enough so they can hear them. This is exactly what hearing aids do.

While otosclerosis can result in a significant hearing loss, it is one of the more correctable or at least treatable of ear diseases. If a person was to be randomly assigned a particular ear disease, they could do a whole lot worse than having otosclerosis.

Meniere's Disease

Meniere's disease is characterized by dizziness, head noises, pressure or fullness in the ear and a fluctuating hearing loss. The disease can develop in both ears, but usually is seen in just one. The dizziness or vertigo goes beyond simple unsteadiness or lightheadedness. Either the person will feel themselves spinning or have the sensation of the room spinning around them. It is not possible to hold the bed tight enough to keep yourself or the room from seeming to spin. The Meniere's attacks come and go. There are good days, weeks or months and bad days, weeks or months. It is impossible to predict when Meniere's will hit or how bad the attack will be. The tinnitus, fullness, and hearing loss are also at their worst during these attacks, but this is often a secondary concern to the dizziness.

Meniere's disease results from a build up of fluid pressure in the balance (vestibular) portion of the inner ear. This extra pressure causes the ear to react as if it were in motion. It sends a message to the brain saying things are spinning around and the brain can't ignore the signals, even if it knows better. There is no cure for Meniere's disease, but it can be controlled. Physicians can prescribe medications to minimize or stop Meniere's attacks by preventing or lessening this extra fluid pressure. Diet and lifestyle changes are also used to reduce the frequency and severity of attacks. Physicians can also prescribe medications to stop or minimize the dizziness during Meniere's attacks. If nausea and vomiting result from the dizziness (as can sometimes happen), medication can be prescribed to deal with this. In severe cases, surgery may be performed to drain off the build up of fluid in the inner ear, sever the nerve pathways that carry the faulty signals from the ear to the brain or remove the balance portion of the ear to prevent the signals from being sent in the first place. More recently, medication is being injected into the middle ear that can destroy the disturbed balance mechanism while preserving hearing. This minimally invasive treatment is often effective and eliminates the need for the more involved surgeries that were the only option just a few years ago.

Once the dizziness is under control, hearing becomes the next major concern for Meniere's patients. Early Meniere's sufferers may have hearing that fluctuates from normal to a mild hearing loss. Long time Meniere's sufferers may have much worse hearing that can still fluctuate. It is not uncommon for both the level and clarity of hearing to fluctuate. This variability makes it very difficult for a person with Meniere's disease to depend on the bad ear. One day they may hear fairly well and the next day hear just awful. Surgery cannot repair this roller coaster of hearing. The best that can be done is to compensate with a hearing aid. Some of the newer programmable or digital hearing aids that can hold multiple memories are most helpful for Meniere's sufferers. The aid can have separately programmed memories for when the hearing is very good, very bad or at a number of points in-between. The user can pick the setting that is best for them on a particular day. Restoring sound to the ear with a hearing aid may also act to lessen the feeling of fullness and to cover up the tinnitus.

Meniere's is pretty far up on the yuck meter of ear diseases. Living with this disease can be a long hard road. But, it can usually be controlled or at least treated so that a person can lead a normal life.

Acoustic Neuroma

An acoustic neuroma is a slow growing tumor that develops on the hearing nerve leading between the inner ear and brain. Although rare, they make up perhaps 5 to 10% of all brain tumors. This kind of growth is not usually malignant, so it does not spread to other parts of the body and cause problems there. The danger from an acoustic neuroma is that there is very limited space within the skull for it to grow. Whatever direction it may expand, it will squish something. Given enough time, it may find something vital (possibly the brain itself). An acoustic neuroma is one of the few ear problems that can be fatal if ignored.

An acoustic neuroma can produce a variety of symptoms. It rarely sneaks up without at least some warning. One of the first symptoms may be tinnitus in the affected ear. This is caused by the tumor putting pressure on and damaging the nerve leading from the ear to the brain. Hearing loss and a sensation of pressure may also result. A hearing loss that is present in only one ear, a hearing loss that is greater in one ear than the other, or tinnitus that is present in only one ear act as a glowing beacon to alarm ear professionals that an acoustic neuroma is a possibility and needs to be identified or ruled out. Sudden hearing loss and dizziness are other possible symptoms. The majority of the time, these symptoms will be diagnosed as another less serious pathology (nerve damage in the inner ear, etc.). However, the stakes are too high not to check every suspected case.

For an ear doctor or audiologist, the patient history and hearing test are the first clues there may be a problem. Other in-office tests may be performed to try to identify the symptoms as being due to another cause. When there is high suspicion of a tumor or it cannot effectively be ruled out with simple tests, magnetic resonance imaging (MRI) serves as the definitive test. An MRI uses magnetic waves to take pictures of what is actually going on with the hearing nerve. The test does not tell anything about hearing, but if there is a tumor on the hearing nerve, it will show it. While very effective, conventional MRI is also very expensive. Fortunately, a newer, faster and cheaper version of the MRI (the Fast Spin MRI) is dramatically lowering costs.

If a tumor is found, surgical removal is the best possible treatment. If the tumor is small, it can sometimes be removed without any further damage to the hearing. If the tumor is larger, the hearing and balance mechanism for that ear may need to be sacrificed in order to remove all of the tumor. The larger the tumor, the greater the risk. As with any other major surgery, there is the possibility of complications.

Although an acoustic neuroma may potentially be the most life threatening of ear problems, it can usually be successfully removed. If completely removed, it is unlikely to return. Yearly MRI tests are performed for a time after surgery just to be sure everything looks OK. Normally it does. While they would not choose to have an acoustic neuroma, people with other, more chronic ear problems only dream of such closure.

Presbycusis

Presbycusis is the diagnosis reserved for nerve hearing losses that are attributed to aging. Regardless of what the name implies, this affliction is not limited only to Presbyterians. It affects about one in four adults by the age of 65 no matter what their religion. Presbycusis is even more likely to be seen in older individuals. The majority of the time, both ears are affected equally.

Presbycusis is not a single disease process. It encompasses a number of different changes that can take place in an older ear as it wears out. Since presbycusis is caused by a number of different inner ear problems, it only follows that hearing losses attributed to presbycusis will not all look alike.

It is not possible to medically or surgically fix hearing losses due to presbycusis. The parts involved are to one extent or another, just worn out. And, unfortunately, we do not know how to make new ones. Regardless of this, it

92

should not be assumed that just because a person is old, their hearing loss is due to presbycusis. There are a number of other ear diseases that can affect the hearing of seniors. Some of these can be corrected through medication or surgery, while others may need treatment to prevent or minimize further loss of hearing.

It is possible to help compensate for presbycusis-related hearing losses through the use of hearing aids. The person may not hear like they did when they were a kid, but they will hear better with than without the hearing aids. Even if a person has only fair or poor word understanding, hearing aids can still be helpful. They will make sound loud enough to have a good chance to make out what is said. Without them, a person might be unaware that anyone was speaking or hear the speaker so softly as to have no chance. People with presbycusis will not all perform equally well with hearing aids due to the diversity in their underlying hearing losses. What is important, is that most can perform better with hearing aids. It may not be possible to fix the problem, but it is possible to help compensate for it.

Sudden Hearing Loss

Sudden hearing loss refers to an abrupt drop in hearing of usually unknown etiology (cause). It is not one specific disease, but rather, a diagnosis descriptive of what has happened. A person may wake up one morning to find that they can no longer hear out of one of their ears. Another person may be reading the newspaper in the evening, hear a loud ping or roaring and then realize that the hearing is gone. One of the ways to identify a person with sudden hearing loss is that they can say exactly when they lost their hearing. This is not the person who has had hearing problems off and on for years and then "suddenly" decided that their hearing loss was bothering them. Their hearing suddenly went away. Another characteristic that identifies someone with a sudden hearing loss is how "freaked out" they are by it. Due to the abruptness of the problem, these people often envision the worst. If they could be fine one day and deaf the next, what could tomorrow bring?

Not all hearing losses that occur abruptly are diagnosed as a sudden hearing loss. If the hearing had dropped because of earwax, the diagnosis would be earwax. Following wax removal, the diagnosis might be normal hearing. If the hearing was lost because of a bad car accident, the diagnosis would be trauma. The diagnosis would be otitis media if the cause was infection or fluid in the middle ear. When the cause is known, the hearing loss is identified by what caused it, rather than fooling around and describing that it was sudden.

The vast majority of the time a sudden hearing loss strikes only in one ear. In the few cases where it does occur in both ears, it will usually happen simultaneously or only a day or two following the drop in the first ear. However, when a sudden hearing loss occurs in one ear, it is highly unlikely for the same thing to happen to the other ear months or years later. The opposite ear remains normal. The degree of nerve hearing loss in the affected ear can range from mild to a total hearing loss. The clarity of hearing can also be affected to varying degrees.

Sudden hearing losses are sometimes thought to be caused by a blockage of the blood supply to the ear, but more often by a virus that attacks the inner ear directly. Usually, it is never known whether a particular sudden hearing loss was caused by a blockage, virus or some other agent. Regardless of this, every sudden hearing loss needs to be checked out. A tumor on the hearing nerve (acoustic neuroma) can cause these same symptoms and lead to even worse problems if left untreated. The worries of the more "freaked out" sudden hearing loss sufferers are not always unfounded.

Although a sudden hearing loss affects the hearing nerves suggesting that the loss would be permanent, in about half of the cases the hearing improves or returns to normal, even without treatment. The odds are a little better for mild losses and worse for more severe losses. It may be that a blockage only starved (not killed) the hearing nerves of oxygen and given time, they recover. Alternately, a virus might suppress the ability of the hearing nerves to work properly, but given time, they improve or return to normal. Medical treatment has been reported to further improve this 50% chance for hearing return by reducing any possible swelling within or surrounding the ear. The sooner treatment is begun following the onset of hearing loss, the greater the chance for hearing recovery.

Anyone experiencing a sudden hearing loss should see an ear doctor as soon as possible. More serious or related problems can be ruled out and treatment can quickly be started to maximize the chance for hearing return. All this having been done, those with a sudden hearing loss in only one ear (the majority) can rest assured that the chance for the same thing happening to the other ear is very remote.

Auditory Processing Disorders

When sounds that are so meticulously picked up, transmitted through and coded by the ear, are lost, distorted or in some other way trashed within the brain, a person can be considered to have an auditory processing disorder. This is not really a disease so much as a matter of less than optimal function. Technically, this is not a hearing loss. These people can hear soft sounds and repeat simple words. Their problems begin when the listening gets tough, such as hearing in background noise or when there are several people talking. Some people naturally process sounds a little better or worse than others. There are also medical conditions (stroke, the results of trauma, etc.) that can limit the brain's ability to process and effectively make use of sound. A person is not considered to have an auditory processing disorder unless they do much worse than average with their understanding of

95

words. There is a wide range that is considered normal, these people are way outside.

To the casual observer, a person with an auditory processing disorder may appear to have a hearing loss. They may misunderstand what is said or ask for things to be repeated. They may also have difficulty following directions, become distracted in background noise or fail to respond appropriately to what is said. It can also appear that they are just not too bright.

The first step in dealing with a person having an auditory processing disorder is to recognize that this is the underlying problem. The second step is to treat any developmental or educational delays resulting from the disorder. Finally, the third step is to develop strategies that help to compensate.

A full hearing evaluation is performed first to rule out hearing loss as the cause of the problem. The symptoms that cause most people to suspect an auditory processing disorder are usually due to an actual hearing loss, rather than a processing disorder. A person has to be able to hear a sound for them to have a chance to process it. Once a hearing loss has been ruled out, there are a number of different tests of auditory processing. Most focus on recognizing or repeating words that have in some way been made more difficult to hear. The words might be couched in a background of people talking or some other noise. The words can also be distorted in some way. The person listens to a tape of this messed up speech and tries to repeat what is being said. They may also be required to repeat it back in some specific order, making things even more difficult. People with auditory processing disorders may do very well in easy listening situations, but they do just awful once things get tougher. Although not very exciting, these and other tests of auditory processing are painless and accurate.

Children with auditory processing disorders can have delayed speech or language problems due to the incoming speech signal being distorted or lost amidst other sounds.

Speech and language therapy is sometimes needed to overcome existing delays and to keep the child functioning at age appropriate levels. Schoolwork and other learning can also be affected. Tutoring and individualized educational plans may additionally be needed to remediate educational delays and to keep things on track.

While it is not possible in most cases to eliminate an auditory processing problem, it is possible to compensate for it. Reducing background noise and other distractions to create an easier listening situation will help most people with auditory processing disorders. Using visual information (graphs, charts, pictures etc.) in combination with what is being said is also helpful. Getting it in writing is the biggest help. Students can read the textbook or copy a classmate's notes. Working people can get a list of the day's tasks or the steps to do a task rather than relying on what was heard or possibly misheard. An audiologist, speech pathologist, psychologist or educational specialist can help an individual develop effective compensatory strategies.

Nonorganic Hearing Loss

It should not be too surprising that in addition to those people who have a hearing loss but would rather not, there are people without a hearing loss that would rather give the impression that they did. There are a few people who actually want a hearing loss. These are usually children who do not understand the down side to their wish or adults who would be found a few marbles short should anyone go to the trouble to count. However, most of the time, people trying to give the impression of a hearing loss (faking) are doing so for distinct personal or financial reasons.

Children fake a hearing loss for a number of reasons. The most common is to get attention or to get out of school. Since the general expectation is for children to hear well, everyone is surprised and concerned if a child appears to have a hearing problem or reports not hearing well. The child immediately becomes the center of attention and will sometimes go to great lengths to stay there. A more goal-oriented reason for faking a hearing loss is to get out of school or schoolwork. It is not all that uncommon to see a normally hearing child who has been out or school for a few days or even a couple weeks because they were faking a hearing loss. The parents have no way of knowing that the hearing loss is fictitious. During the time it took the parents to find the proper professionals to check this out, the child had their own personal little vacation. This imaginary hearing loss could also (at least for a while) excuse prior grades and distance them from any personal problems at school. This behavior is most frequently seen in teenagers and usually does not represent a deep seated psychological problem.

The primary reason adults fake a hearing loss is for money. They feel that there may be gold in that there imaginary hearing loss. They may have worked around noise or have been involved in some form of an accident (car wreck, falling on ice, being hit in the head, etc.) and envisioned an imaginary hearing loss as the road to fabulous wealth and fortune. Others may seek the classification of being handicapped in order to obtain life long disability payments. There are a few adults who will fake a hearing loss for attention or for other reasons, but normally it is for the money.

Faking a hearing loss is not reserved only for those with normal hearing. Possibly the most common type of faking takes the form of exaggerating a hearing loss. A person with a mild hearing loss may act like they have a slightly worse or much worse hearing loss. A person with a severe hearing loss may act like they hear nothing at all. This form of faking is fairly common when reimbursement for hearing loss is based on its severity. A bigger loss means more money.

Regardless of the underlying reason for a person faking a hearing loss, their chance of success is just about zero. A full hearing evaluation is made up of several distinct parts that have to agree with each other. The separate tests form certain patterns that either do or do not make sense. A well trained and experienced ear professional will recognize normal patterns from those that would indicate an imaginary or exaggerated hearing loss. If the person continues to respond this way after having been talked to and given a second chance, then the irregularities that confirm faking are documented. At this point, other tests that do not require truthful responses to determine hearing may also be performed (with or without the patient's knowledge). It may not always be possible to determine the exact hearing level of someone faking or exaggerating a hearing loss, but it is almost always possible to determine when a person is faking.

If a person is considering the use of an imaginary ailment to finance the rest of their life, hearing loss is not the best way to go. People faking a hearing loss are unlikely to get away with it. People exaggerating a hearing loss will be classified as faking and risk losing any compensation for the hearing loss they do have. Even if people could get away with faking a hearing loss, compared to other things, hearing loss does not pay that well anyway.

Chapter Six: Augmenting Your Hearing

Lip-Reading

The first way to help compensate for a hearing loss or to augment normal hearing in difficult listening situations is to lip-read. Everyone does this to one extent or another. Some will lip-read by staring at others with such intensity as to give them a complex. Others will hardly seem to watch at all, but still pick up lip-reading cues. We have all clearly understood the unheard exclamation of a football coach when one of his players fumbles the football or the silent words of a golfer who just missed a simple putt. We do not always need to hear it. The combination of knowing what a person is likely to say in a particular situation as well as seeing their body language and lip movements is enough to convey the message. Even people who deny any lip-reading ability whatsoever can do this to some extent.

Although lip-reading can be very helpful, it is not possible to understand everything that is said by lip-reading alone. There are several different speech sounds that are made with the lips in the same position. For instance, the letters "p", "b" and "m" are visually identical. To know which was said, it is either necessary to hear the sound or to discern it from the context of the sentence.

While not perfect, lip-reading can work very well to fill in some of the speech sounds missed due to a hearing loss or difficult listening environment. The majority of the time when speech is not clearly understood, people still hear most of it and almost always have some idea as to the context of what is being said. Adding the visual cues from lip-reading can fill in the gaps so that little is misunderstood. Some people will do this naturally, while others need to take classes through a speech or hearing professional to become proficient in lip-reading. To succeed, it is important to get into a position where you can see the person talking and watch their face. It is not necessary to stare until you have no more friends. Casually watching is enough most of the time. People with beards or mustaches will be more difficult to lip-read as will those individuals who talk without ever seeming to move their mouth. Fortunately, most people are not furry and actually do move their mouth when talking, so lip-reading can be used. It does not replace hearing, but does help to augment it.

Listening Strategies

Hearing can be more than happenstance. Like in a chess game, one is more likely to win if they have a well thought out strategy. Unlike chess, in the hearing world, it is possible to change many of the rules to give yourself an advantage. In other words, to a large extent, you can cheat.

Planning to hear better does not have to be difficult. The first step is to recognize the specific situations that cause a problem. The second step is to change each situation in some way to make it easier. In the majority of cases the goals will be to increase the loudness of the person speaking or to limit other sounds that may be covering them up. Accomplishing these goals will be different in each situation. This is why situation specific strategies are needed. There is an old adage that people do not plan to fail. They fail to plan. Rather than failing to hear, people can plan to hear. Below are some examples:

Problem: I can't hear the sermon at church because the pastor is soft spoken.

Strategy: Sitting in a different seat would be the first thing to try. Moving closer to the pastor or closer to a speaker if the church has a sound system could help. Additionally, due to peculiarities in the acoustics of some rooms, the sound can be focused toward or away from a particular place. Move around to see if there is a place you can hear better. Asking that the pastor speak louder or that the sound system be turned louder would also be an option. If embarrassed to try the direct approach to get the pastor to talk louder, less direct approaches are also possible. You could mention to the pastor or church council how concerned you are that 104 year old Mrs. Smith (fill in your local equivalent) may not be able to hear the service. Since Mrs. Smith has always been very kind and polite and would never complain even if she couldn't hear, the pastor or council might turn up the sound system a little just in case.

Problem: I can't hear other people in the car.

Strategy: Reduce as much of the noise inside the car as possible. Turn down the radio, roll up the window, drive more slowly or on smoother roads. However, having done all of this, some cars will still be very loud inside making it difficult to hear. In these cases, a different car might be the best solution. Car dealers sometimes have ratings of the interior noise levels for the cars they sell. If you need a very quiet car, these can be used for comparisons.

Problem: I can't hear the television in the living room when the air conditioner is running.

Strategy: Arrange the room so you sit closer to the television and as far away from the air conditioner as possible. If you wish to sit further from the television, then an auxiliary speaker(s) placed near you would help. Headphones connected to the television would be another option.

Problem: I can't hear my companion in Finicky Fred's restaurant because of the background music and other people talking.

Strategy: Find an area away from the speakers where the music is softer. This may be a corner or a separate room which does not have speakers. Sitting with your back to a wall gets rid of 1/2 the noise around you. Eating at off-hours is also a possibility. The restaurant will be quieter due to fewer people talking. The background music will likely be turned softer since it will not need to be so loud to be heard. Going to a different, quieter restaurant would be another possibility. A more familiar possibility would be to invite your friend to dinner at your home. This would give things a personal touch and you would have greater control of the surrounding sounds.

Problem: I can't hear people I can't see.

Strategy: As previously noted, most people lip-read at least a little bit whether they realize it or not. Moving to a position where you can see the person talking is often of help if you can't quite hear everything that is being said. This may include moving closer to the front in a theater or church. It may also mean buying a larger television so it is easier to see the people talking. Consciously or subconsciously, you'll pick up more of what is being said.

Problem: I can't hear the driver when riding in the car, but I can hear the passenger when I am driving, due to better hearing in the right ear.

Strategy: The most direct solution would be to tell the person you are with that you hear better when you drive. A less direct solution would be to say that you prefer to drive. For the truly hard to convince, tell them you get car sick if you don't drive. On the other hand, if you hear better as a passenger, then you might say that you are tired or prefer to just look out the window.

Problem: I can't hear on the phone.

Strategy: Since the break-up of the phone company a number of years ago, all telephones have not been created equal. It used to be that most phones looked about the same, were made about the same and sounded about the same. Not now. Some phones today are better than they have ever been. Some of the phones out there are junk. The first thing to do if you can't hear on the phone is to try another one. If you can find a phone on which you hear well, then the best strategy is to buy one just like it. While convenient, cordless phones are often not the best choice for people with hearing problems due to radio interference reducing the sound quality. If conventional phones aren't good enough, there are ones made specifically for people with hearing problems. The volume on these phones (and sometimes the pitch) can be adjusted to the level that is best for the person. If all of the phones in the house are about the same, pick the one in the quietest room. Conversely, if the person on the other end of the phone is in a noisy room, it will be more difficult to hear them. Convince them to move to a phone in a quieter room. In the not too distant future, phones will have video in addition to audio. You will be able to see and lip-read the person you are talking to. An early version of this is available now to those who make calls through the computer internet. It is still a little bit awkward, but stands to revolutionize how we make phone calls.

Problem: I can't hear the person I'm with when I do _____ .

Strategy: Don't do _____ . If you can't hear during business lunches at the bar across the street from your office, switch the business lunches to a quieter restaurant or to a private conference room. If you can't hear your spouse while the water is running in the sink, talk to them before or after doing the dishes. If you can't hear on your car phone while driving 70 mph on the interstate, talk to the person later or pull off at a rest stop so you will be able to hear without all the road noise. You can still have business lunches, talk to your spouse and use the car phone. You just may need to plan a little bit how to do these things effectively.

Acoustics

We have just discussed strategies to hear better, now it is necessary to take a closer look at the places where we are trying to hear. This is often overlooked when people discuss hearing or hearing problems. Background noise, mumbling, talking soft, not speaking clearly or speaking with a foreign accent, serve as the usual suspects when something is misheard. Few suspect that the acoustics of their physical surroundings might be the culprit.

Acoustics could generally be defined as the study or science of sound. Of concern here is how the physical characteristics of a room, or the arrangement of things within a room, serve to enhance or interfere with what a person is trying to hear. Although it sounds simple, this is all controlled by a number of physical laws that could give nightmares to anyone other than a physicist. What are the characteristics of the sound? What direction is it coming from? Where does it need to go? Will the floors, walls and ceiling reflect or absorb the sound? Where will they reflect it? How will other sounds interact with it? The questions go on and on. Fortunately, it is possible to make use of some of the basic laws of acoustics without having to resort to slide rules, calculators or computers.

The simplest rule of acoustics is that as we double the distance from a sound, we reduce its power by half. Put more simply, we hear things that are close better than things that are far away. A second general rule is that sound reflects better off surfaces that are hard and smooth than surfaces that are porous and rough. Related to this second rule is that reflected sound can cover up what a person is trying to hear.

We all know that it is easier to hear things that are close than things that are far away. However, in our everyday lives, we often forget about or fail to make use of this knowledge. We might sit right next to a furnace vent and be surprised we hear this better than the television across the room. We might not even think to put our favorite chair closer to the television. Changing the seating arrangement in a business meeting to be closer to the most soft spoken or most important person would effectively make them louder than the ambient room noise. Similarly, a teacher may find that they are having difficulty understanding the quietest children in class. Instead of repeatedly asking these children to talk louder, it might be easier and work every bit as well to seat them at the front of the class. If it is possible to get closer to what you are trying to hear, in most situations, you are likely to hear it better.

Beyond simply arranging things within a room, it is also helpful to take a good look at the room itself. Specialists can be called in to maximize building acoustics. This is often done when theaters or churches are constructed. However, more often, cost effective construction outweighs concerns about acoustics. It is up to the people who end up living and working in these buildings to worry about the acoustics.

One of the most commonly committed acoustical sins is to create a large room with hard, flat, reflective surfaces. Sounds made by everyone and everything within the room just bounce around between the walls, floor and ceiling. We have all experienced this in a meeting room, classroom or restaurant. The ambient noise covers up everything. This is why schools will often carpet over perfectly good wood or tile floors. The carpet absorbs sound. Acoustic ceiling tiles, curtains or wall hangings can do the same thing. The sound coming to us directly from the person talking is not lessened by these materials. It is only the reflection or echo from these and other sounds that are eliminated.

The smaller rooms in the average house are less prone to problems from reflected sound. This is primarily because fewer people will fit and there are less things to make noise. This does not mean, however, that private residences do not have acoustical problems. In rooms with hardwood floors, drywall or plaster ceilings and walls, even limited sources of sound can add up to distracting levels. Stray sound from the television, refrigerator, dishwasher, furnace, washer, dryer and other household appliances can all limit what we are trying to hear. Decorating with materials to absorb some of these unwanted sounds is worthwhile from more than an aesthetic point of view. Having a conversation or listening to the television will be easier without all of the reflected sound competing with or covering up what you want to hear.

All of the above assumes that the sound a person is trying to hear (person talking, television, radio, etc.) is coming directly at them. If the sound initially starts out in another direction and has to bounce off a wall to reach the listener, much of it will be lost or deflected in the wrong direction. Arranging furniture so people can face each other greatly enhances understandability. Likewise, a television set with the speaker(s) in front directly facing the listener will usually be easier to understand than a monitor type television where the speaker(s) are facing sideways.

Arranging the acoustics of a room to favor the listener does not have to be treated like rocket science. By getting close, directing the sound to the listener and using materials to limit or absorb ambient noise, it is possible to greatly improve what is heard.

Assistive Listening Devices

In addition to changing how we plan to hear and where we plan to hear, there are also a number of devices that can be useful when we need to hear better. Most of these are designed to help with a specific listening problem such as talking on the phone or hearing the television. In fact, a person who only has trouble hearing in one or two specific situations is sometimes better served by one of these devices than with hearing aids. However, many assistive listening devices can be used with or are specifically designed to be used with hearing aids.

The first kind of these assistive devices can be termed "alerting devices". They make it easier to hear or be aware of signals or alarms. These might include extra loud ringers or bells for telephones, alarm clocks, door bells and smoke or fire alarms. A hearing impaired person cannot act on a problem if they are not aware of it. For those with very severe hearing losses, flashing lights are available as the signal for various alarms. Because a sleeping person would be unlikely to see a flashing light, vibrating alarm clocks are made for the hearing impaired. Rather than setting the clock on a counter or bed side table, a person takes it to bed with them and is vibrated awake. There are also vibrating pocket pagers.

Hearing on the phone is another area people often need assistance. Without lip-reading, they have to depend exclusively on what they hear and what they can pick up from the context of the conversation. The simplest solution is often to buy a telephone with a volume control that can be adjusted to whatever level is needed. There are also portable amplifiers made that can fit over the earpiece of many phones. A telecoil is the best bet for a person who uses a hearing aid (discussed later). For those who need to communicate with a phone but have too little hearing to use one, there are telephone typewriters. Each of these has a typewriter keyboard and a small display screen. A person may type and read, rather than talk. E-mail and computer chat rooms are also becoming recognized as an alternative way for hearing impaired people to communicate.

Another form of assistive listening device works to overcome long distances or poor acoustics. Most of these place a microphone very close to the person talking and then transmit the sound (through wires, radio or light waves) directly to the listener. This keeps other sounds between the talker and listener from interfering. There are many versions of this device. One of the simplest transmits sound from a television across the room to the person watching. The person can either listen through headphones or some will work with hearing aids. Versions of this device have also been created to work in schools, churches, movie theaters and other public buildings. In each case, the device focuses on what the person wants or needs to hear and keeps the surrounding sounds of the other students, congregation or theater goers from getting in the way.

These are a few examples of assistive listening devices. There are many more. Some are brand new and pretty much unknown to the general public, while others have become so common place (like closed captioning for television) that we hardly think about them. When a person has trouble hearing in a few specific situations, there is a good chance that they are not the first one with this problem. Someone may already have created just the gizmo to help in their specific case. An audiologist would be able to provide information on what is available.

Chapter Seven: Hearing Aids

Do I Need Hearing Aids?

Deciding whether a person needs hearing aids can have as much to do with how we define "need" as with the amount of hearing loss. If we define needing hearing aids as only including those who could not possibly live without them, then very few people need hearing aids. Hearing impaired people who do not wear hearing aids rarely explode, dissolve or spontaneously combust. Aside from the risk of being run over by an unheard plane, train or automobile, failing to wear hearing aids is not usually fatal. Some may even take this as proof that they do not need hearing aids. Insurance companies often conclude that they do not need to cover hearing aids for their policy holders since hearing loss is not life threatening. If we widen our view to define the need for hearing aids as making it possible for people to live happier, fuller or more productive lives, then many more need hearing aids. The latter is closer to the public definition of need.

The amount of hearing loss generally accepted as indicating the need for hearing aids is about 30% or greater. Since most people talk at a moderately loud level, small hearing losses are less likely to affect speech understanding and may go unnoticed. Once a hearing loss reaches about 30%, people have difficulty understanding someone who is soft spoken and begin having difficulty with speech at normal conversational levels. Difficult listening demands would necessitate hearing aids sooner. Business executives, lawyers, and students would need hearing aids for much smaller losses because they cannot afford to misunderstand anything being said. Someone with less difficult listening demands might not need hearing aids until their loss is greater. A retired person living alone could always turn the television, radio or telephone louder.

Regardless of the numbers, people usually judge their need for hearing aids on the basis of whether they feel they hear well enough in most situations. If a person thinks they do well in most situations, they will be unlikely to wear hearing aids. Even if they hear better with hearing aids, they may still not wear them if there is no perceived need. While they might not like to admit it, most people know when their hearing gets bad enough that they need help. They simply reach a point where they are missing too many of the things they need or want to hear. It is only when they reach this point that they become motivated to see what can be done about it.

Almost anyone with any amount of hearing loss could hear better with hearing aids. Yet for people with very small hearing losses, there may be little perceived improvement since they already hear most of the things they need to. Many of the severe or profoundly hearing impaired in the deaf community accept or have come to accept not being able to hear as normal and live their lives quite happily that way. They do not want hearing aids even if they could hear better with them. However, for the majority of hearing impaired people who fall between these slight and profound hearing losses, the need for and potential benefit from hearing aids increase with larger hearing losses and more difficult listening demands. The proper question for these individuals is not whether they need or can live without hearing aids, but rather, whether they could live better with them.

What Hearing Aids Do

Hearing aids work by making the sounds a person can't hear louder. The goal is not to make all sounds louder, only the pitches where there is hearing loss. The hearing aids for a person with a high-pitched hearing loss will emphasize (boost) high-pitched sounds. The hearing aids for a person with a low-pitched hearing loss will emphasize low pitched sounds. A person with a hearing loss across all pitches will need hearing aids that makes all pitches louder. Because of these differences in hearing, hearing aids have to be designed or adjusted differently for each individual's specific hearing loss.

In addition to the pitch of a person's hearing loss dictating the design of a hearing aid, the amount of hearing loss also has to be taken into account. People with large hearing losses need powerful hearing aids. People with smaller losses need less power. For those with a greater degree of hearing loss at some pitches than others, the hearing aid(s) needs to be capable of different amounts of power at different pitches.

Once we take into account the degree of hearing loss across the pitches, we must also consider an individual's sensitivity to loud sounds. A person with hearing loss can be just as sensitive or even more sensitive to loud sounds than a person with normal hearing. Consider what happens when a person with normal hearing and a person with a severe hearing loss listen to a radio with 10 volume settings. For the normal hearing person, volume setting 1 would be very soft, 2 and 3 would be a little louder but still soft, 4, 5 and 6 would be comfortable, 7 and 8 would be loud, 9 would be very loud and 10 would be uncomfortably loud. The person with a severe hearing loss would not hear volume settings 1 through 6. Volume settings 7 and 8 would be fairly soft, 9 would be comfortably loud and 10 would be uncomfortably loud. The hearing impaired person could perceive volume setting 10 just as loud as a person with normal hearing. Further, they would experience this increase in volume more abruptly, rather than gradually as a normal hearing person would. This is why a hearing impaired person might ask someone to speak up and then complain that they are yelling when they have only increased the volume of their voice a small amount. Because of this, it is not unusual for it to take repeated fine tuning before hearing aids can be adjusted loud enough to hear without becoming uncomfortably loud.

Traditionally, the goal in fitting hearing aids has been to compensate for about half of the hearing a person has lost. A 50% hearing loss would be improved to 25%, or an 80% loss

114

to 40% etc. The hearing aid does this by increasing the loudness of sounds by a certain amount (or within a certain range, for hearing aids with an adjustable volume control). Since both loud and soft sounds are increased by the same amount, it is only possible to compensate for so much hearing loss before loud sounds become uncomfortably loud. While hearing aids may limit their maximum loudness, this level usually needs to be set fairly high so that important loud sounds (tires screeching, a fire alarm etc.) are not blocked out. If we apply this kind of hearing aid (linear technology with output limiting) to our previous radio example, the person will hear more, but still not everything. Rather than hearing from 7 to 10 on the radio volume control, they would now be able to hear from 3 1/2 to 10. Setting 4 would be very soft, settings 5 and 6 comfortable, and 7 through 10 loud and bordering on uncomfortable. The person would still not hear the radio when it was turned soft (below setting 3 1/2). If a person started with a smaller hearing loss, it would be possible to hear softer sounds, but they would still reach a point where loud sounds limited how much they could stand to turn up their hearing aid(s).

A newer approach being made possible by technological advances is to take the full range of sounds audible to a person with normal hearing and to compress them into a loudness range that is perceptible and comfortable for a hearing impaired person. Under this strategy, soft and loud sounds are not boosted equally. Very soft sounds may be given a great deal of boost to make them hearable while louder sounds are given very little boost, so they do not become too loud. If done correctly, the hearing aid wearer will have a normal perception of increasing loudness with increases in volume. For our severely hearing impaired person who only hears from 7 to 10 on the radio volume control, the sound coming out of the radio at volume setting 1 would be boosted up to a loudness equivalent to volume 7. The sound at volume setting 2 would be boosted up to a loudness

115

equivalent of 7 1/3. Volume 3 would become 7 2/3, volume 4 would become 8, volume 5 would become 8 1/3, volume 6 would become 8 2/3, volume 7 would become 9, volume 8 would become 9 1/3, volume 9 would become 9 2/3 and volume 10 would remain as volume 10. To the hearing impaired person, it would sound like they had the full 10 settings on their volume control. While this may sound relatively easy, in practice, it is frighteningly difficult. Because hearing impaired people usually have differing hearing losses and differing sensitivity to loud sounds with each pitch, the hearing aid would need to be capable of making these volume conversions separately at each individual pitch from 20 - 20,000 CPS. Today's technology is good, but it is not that good. Currently these volume conversions can be done across a few separate bands, but not for every conceivable pitch. Consequently, the goal of taking all sound and compressing it into an range audible for a hearing impaired person while maintaining the perception of normal loudness growth is seldom perfectly achieved.

There is not complete agreement between hearing care professionals as to which of these or other more exotic strategies might be best, or how to implement them. This can sometimes result in differing hearing aid recommendations for the same person or in alternative hearing aid strategies being tried if the first strategy was unsuccessful. As a general rule, experienced hearing aid users prefer to stay with traditional hearing aids because this is what they are used to. Once they get used to the loudness of a traditional fitting, other strategies are likely to sound soft, creating the perception they are not hearing. Either strategy could be used with new hearing aid users. All of the current hearing aid strategies will help a hearing impaired person hear better, but the jury is still out whether one fitting strategy has a clear advantage over another.

Will Hearing Aids Hurt My Hearing Or Cause Me To Become Dependent?

A frequently asked question is whether hearing aids will damage the ears or cause further hearing loss. This is a valid question. Since loud sounds can damage hearing and hearing aids work by making sounds louder, it only follows that hearing aids could damage hearing. In some cases this can be true. To make it possible for a person with a severe or profound hearing loss to hear, it may be necessary to make the sounds so loud that they could damage a person's hearing over time. However, this is usually undertaken as a rational and informed choice, since these people cannot hear much of anything without the hearing aids. Fortunately, the majority of hearing impaired people have a much milder loss and do not need so much volume. They can hear just fine without their hearing aids having to become uncomfortably or dangerously loud. In fact, the hearing aids can be designed to stay within safe levels that pose no threat to the person's remaining hearing, even when they are surrounded by sounds that are fairly loud. For the vast majority of the hearing impaired, hearing aids pose little or no risk to a person's remaining hearing.

A related concern is whether a person will become dependent on hearing aids. Those who are able to get by in most situations may be hesitant to try hearing aids if they believe they may end up needing them all the time. The truth, even if unsettling, is that the goal is to end up feeling the need for them. Once a person gets used to wearing hearing aids, they also get used to living again in a world of sound. After a few months of hearing aid use, some will feel that their hearing has worsened. However, it is not that the hearing has changed, but rather, that they now recognize the things that they cannot hear without their hearing aids. They do not end up needing the hearing aids more, but wanting the hearing aids more. New hearing aid users may see this like sitting in a wheelchair a couple of times and then finding out that they can no longer walk. However, wearing hearing aids is not like this at all. They do not make a person handicapped or cause them to stop hearing. It allows them to hear better and do more.

Someone with marginal vision might worry they could become dependent on glasses or contact lenses to see better. But, the majority choose to see and do not dwell on this. Life is easier and fuller when we do not have to squint, when we can read type smaller than 1/4 inch and when trees have individual leaves as opposed to one giant green blur. Life is also simpler and fuller when we can hear. It is not that a person becomes dependent on hearing aids. They become dependent on hearing.

One Hearing Aid Or Two

Upon deciding that they really need amplification to hear, most peoples' first question is whether they need one or two hearing aids. The simple answer is usually that they need one to hear, but would hear better with two. The problem with one aid is that if the aided ear misses what is said, the person may be out of luck because the hearing in the other ear may not be good enough to help. A hearing aid in the opposite ear could have picked up what was missed. Matters are further confounded by the brain being designed to make use of sounds coming from each ear. In difficult listening situations, the brain compares what one ear hears with what the other ear hears and uses this to help pick out one voice from another or what someone is saying in various background noises. With only one hearing aid, this is much more difficult.

A good analogy exists for the choice between one or two hearing aids. The analogy is a monocle vs. eye glasses. A visually impaired person will see better with a monocle than without. They will be able to read, look around and not bump into too many things when afoot. The problem is that a monocle cannot provide depth perception or stereoscopic vision. Two eyes are needed for this. Similarly, a person can hear with one hearing aid, but they will have difficulty telling from what direction sounds are coming. There will also be less of a sense of depth. The sounds may seem to live in the hearing aid, instead of in the outside world. Two ears are needed for the spatial orientation of sounds. Considering all of this, it is somewhat surprising that some insurance plans will provide reimbursement for eye glasses but only pay for one hearing aid. They consider each eye important, but only one ear. We feel it is important to point this out, but do so with a certain degree of trepidation lest insurance carriers conclude that if they could get away with correcting the hearing in only one ear, the second lens in a pair of eye glasses might also be superfluous and not deserve reimbursement. If this does happen, monocles may be poised for a comeback.

One of the best arguments for two hearing aids is that they sound more natural than just one. The brain is used to hearing in stereo. If we give it a monaural (one ear) signal, it will always sound a little bit artificial or incomplete. The brain adds together the sound from both ears. This means that a person wearing two hearing aids will need a little bit less power in each, than if they were wearing just one. The lower hearing aid gain results in a more natural sound and less chance for hearing aid feedback (whistling).

While two hearing aids are best, there are valid reasons to buy only one. The most common reason is cost. One hearing aid is expensive. Two are twice as much. People who are on a fixed income or have limited resources may be hard pressed to afford even one. The question can become: This is all I can afford, what is my best option? For many, the best option may be to buy two of the less expensive hearing aids available (last year's model, circuitry, etc.) rather than one fancy one. These usually work just fine and let the person hear in stereo. Other people can afford two hearing aids, but can only use one. A person with a hearing loss in one ear and normal hearing in the other obviously will need only one hearing aid. Conversely, a person with some hearing loss in one ear and a total hearing loss in the other ear will usually find a hearing aid useful in only the better hearing ear. There are also medical conditions (infections, skin problems, etc.) which can preclude hearing aid use in an ear. Finally, after trying hearing aids, there are a few people who prefer the sound of one hearing aid over two (even if they hear better with two). However, these are usually people who started with one hearing aid a number of years ago and have gotten used to hearing this way. When they try a second hearing aid, it sounds different from what they are used to, and they don't like it.

The appropriate question is not whether a person needs one or two hearing aids. It is whether a person would hear better or could do more with one or two hearing aids. The answer to this second question is almost always two. Since hearing aid fitters usually sell their hearing aids with a 30-day trial, a person can try them and find out for themselves whether they do better with one or two. The majority of people who try two, stay with two at the end of their trial, because they really do hear better this way.

Trying Hearing Aids

As just noted, most hearing aid dispensers sell their hearing aids on a 30-day trial basis (this option is law is some states). They will usually require a minimum deposit or even the total cost of the hearing aids up front, but will then refund the money (minus a trial fee) if the hearing aids are returned for any reason within the first month. Each party signs a written contract explaining the terms of the trial. The average trial fee (if a hearing aid is returned) is about 10% of the total price of the hearing aids. If the hearing aids are purchased (kept beyond the 30-day trial), the person pays for the hearing aids. There is no separate fee for the trial.

Trying hearing aids is different from taking a car on a test drive. On a test drive, a person can quickly size up the quality and performance of a car based on their experiences with other cars. People who have not tried hearing aids before are used to hearing with a hearing loss. This is what sounds natural to them. No matter how the hearing aids are adjusted, they will sound strange or different. The 30-day trial allows a person time to begin to adjust to a world of sound and then make a decision as to whether the hearing aids help. For those who have previously worn hearing aids, the trial lets them judge in a variety of settings whether the new hearing aids work as well or better than their previous ones.

If, at the end of the trial period a person feels that the hearing aids are not helping or that they are not going to wear them, they should not keep them. There are too many people who pay a great deal of money for their drawer to have hearing aids. It may be that the fitter can take what was learned from this trial and use it to select different or more exotic hearing aids that would work better. But, this option won't exist if a person's money is tied up in unused hearing aids. After trying hearing aids, some will decide that they are just not ready for them yet. Returning the hearing aids at the end of the trial is also indicated for these people since the aids will probably not be worn. If the hearing loss worsens over time or the person's situation changes such that they need to hear more, then the money refunded from the first set of hearing aids will be available for a new set. This new set will be designed for the person's current hearing levels as opposed to the previous level that they did not feel needed corrected.

In a nutshell: Try before you agree to buy.

Size Matters

While it may not apply to all things, as far as hearing aids go, size matters. Large is not always better and small is not always better. Having the appropriate size is better. Few of us would go to buy eyeglasses and specify how thick we wanted the lenses to be. However, most people are willing to go to a hearing aid fitter and specify what size hearing aid they want without asking if it would be optimal, or even possible.

As a general rule, people with larger hearing losses need larger hearing aids. The increased size allows room for a larger and more powerful battery. The added size also allows room for special circuitry to make more efficient use of the battery's power. Some configurations of hearing loss are very difficult to fit and necessitate a larger hearing aid style to accommodate special circuitry. People with milder hearing losses will usually have a greater choice of hearing aid size. For cosmetic reasons, they will often opt for the smallest hearing aid they can get. In addition to the cosmetic benefit, the smallest hearing aids that go way down in the ear canal have occasionally been reported to sound more natural due to acoustic benefits resulting from their close proximity to the eardrum.

A number of practical considerations also have to be recognized when choosing the style (size) of hearing aid. People with arthritis or poor dexterity will have greater difficulty getting small hearing aids into or out of their ears. Changing the tiny batteries can also be difficult for these people and for anyone with a vision problem. In contrast, completely in the canal hearing aids (the smallest ones) can be the preferred option for people who have to use telephones or headphones that may not be hearing aid compatible. A conventional hearing aid would feedback (whistle) if covered up by headphones. These little ones don't.

Special considerations also have to be made for those wishing to use their hearing aids with the assistive listening devices available in movies, theaters, schools and public buildings. They need a hearing aid large enough to accommodate compatible circuitry. People with chronic ear infections (if they can wear a hearing aid) will often need a larger hearing aid with a vent that allows air into the ear. This is not always practical or even possible with some styles. All these considerations and many, many more have to be taken into account when selecting the size of a hearing aid.

The proper question to ask a hearing aid dispenser is: What size hearing aids would be best suited for my hearing loss and activities? It is best to make use of the training and experience of the hearing aid fitter. If they explain why a particular size of hearing aid would be best given your hearing loss and lifestyle, listen to them. Some hearing aid dispensers will refuse to fit a style that they consider inappropriate for a person. Others will recognize that the fit is not optimal, but still sell the aid with the understanding that it is better than nothing. In each case, no one really wins. In the first case, the person walks away hearing no better than when they went in. In the second case, the person ends up dissatisfied with how they hear and blame the hearing aid dispenser for selling hearing aids that are no good.

The small hearing aids that are now available are viewed as a major advance by people considering hearing aids. They overcome the cosmetic objections seen with larger hearing aids because they are pretty much invisible when in the ears. However, they are not for everyone. A person should primarily be concerned with finding the size of hearing aid that will help them hear best. If they can wear the little ones, that is great. However, hearing well should not be viewed as secondary to cosmetics.

A Volume Control Or No Volume Control, That Is The Question

Each hearing aid (or pair of hearing aids) is specifically designed to help compensate for an individual's unique hearing loss. There is little disagreement that people with severe hearing losses need more power (volume) than people with milder losses. There is also little disagreement that people with high pitched hearing losses need the most volume at the high pitches, while people with other hearing losses need power elsewhere. However, there are two distinct schools of thought regarding whether a hearing aid should or should not have a volume control. These schools are populated by the "volume control people" and the "no volume control people".

Ears do not come with a volume control. We cannot turn up soft sounds or turn down loud sounds. We cannot filter out things we do not like. We hear what we hear. Good, bad or otherwise, this is the way ears are and we are used to it. The "no volume control people" believe it should be the same with hearing aids. The hearing aids should be adjusted to what is optimal for a specific individual and then left alone. How can people get used to them or have things sound normal if the volume is always changing?

The "volume control people" feel that the user should be able to adjust the loudness to what they consider optimal. This allows the wearer to vary how powerful they want the hearing aids to be in different settings. They can turn the hearing aids up to hear a soft whisper or turn them down on a noisy bus. We adjust the volume on our televisions, stereos, alarm clocks and even computers to the level that best suits us. Despite changing the volume, we are used to these devices and are not disoriented by being able to change the volume. Why should hearing aids be any different?

Generally speaking, we would side with the "volume control people." If a person had very poor dexterity and could not adjust the hearing aids or if they were mentally handicapped and could not understand how to work the controls, then we might skip the volume control. For just about everyone else, we would want a volume control. People using hearing aids without an adjustable volume control want them set at a level that will be comfortable in all situations. All too often, this means that the hearing aids are set so low (to prevent them from ever becoming uncomfortably loud) that they are of little benefit. Special circuitry that can limit loud sounds helps, but users may still wind up wanting the hearing aids set at a level much lower than what would be optimal. Some of the more exotic hearing aids are self adjusting. They change the volume themselves, unfortunately, not always to the level the user would choose.

Based on our experience, we feel that it is to the user's advantage to be able to adjust the volume themselves. Aside from letting them optimize how well they can hear in different situations, it also gives them some control over their hearing problem (something that is sorely needed by many people with hearing loss). They can always set the volume control to one level and leave it there if they wish. However, with a volume control, the user has the power to change what they can hear, even if they would only want to change it occasionally.

Remote Control

Now that we have decided that a volume control on a hearing aid might be a good idea, we have to decide whether to get one with a conventional volume control or something more exotic. Most hearing aids come with a small knob or wheel that can be turned to adjust the volume. It's tried and true and works very well. Regardless of this, many hearing aid manufacturers are starting to follow the lead of other consumer electronic devices. Walking across the room to adjust the television is considered old fashioned. We can sit in a chair and adjust the TV, VCR, individual stereo components, or whole house environments (provided a real love affair with gadgets beyond The Clapper) by remote control. Why not remote controls for hearing aids? Believe it or not, they're here.

Even though it might be fun at parties, the reason to have a remote control for hearing aids is not to adjust them from across the room. Rather, the point is to provide the user more control. As hearing aids are made smaller, there is less and less room for the knobs, switches or buttons that have traditionally been used to control them. Remote controls solve this problem. Some are small and simple while others have enough buttons and settings to drive a technophobe screaming into the night. There can be separate settings (memories or programs) for normal listening, listening in different kinds of noise, listening to music, singing in the choir, playing croquet in the yard on a windy day and for all kinds of other normal and not so normal activities. Additionally, the overall volume can often be adjusted from within any of these specific programs to further fine tune things. These individual hearing aid programs do not give a person perfect hearing. But, using a remote control lets the user select the individual program most helpful in a particular situation. It may take a while to learn what works best in a specific situation, but once found, it can be saved for future use. Most of today's remote control hearing aids are programmable and can remember at least a few different programs to select from. Theoretically, there is no limit to the number of programs that could be remembered by a hearing aid. The trick for the user is to remember which button(s) to press for the program they need.

While all of this sounds very nice, we need to ask whether people actually like remote control hearing aids and consider them worth the cost? The answer to this question is a resounding "YES" or a resounding "NO" depending on who is asked. Few people who have tried these gadgets are left undecided about them.

In the "NO" remote control camp are the technophobes who try to cope with the remote, but eventually wind up setting it down next to the VCR blinking 12:00. The vanity and miniaturization people also have a big problem with the remote. Why they ask, would the hearing aid industry go to so much trouble to miniaturize hearing aids and then pair them with a remote control larger than the hearing aids made 25 years ago? People not wanting to carry a remote or not remembering where they might have put their remote, likewise end up as members of this group. However, the majority of people who fall into the "NO" remote control camp do so because adding a remote control also adds to the cost.

At the forefront of the "YES" camp are the people with fluctuating hearing losses. The remote lets them adjust the hearing aid to compensate for however their hearing may change (within reason). Also in the "YES" camp are people who need to hear in quite diverse listening environments. A remote control hearing aid can have separate programs for these different environments. Conventional hearing aids usually cannot. A simple remote control with large buttons can work well for a person with arthritis or dexterity problems. This ease of use can make these people remote control hearing aid converts. Gadget people, of course, would also fall into the "YES" group. They consider remote control hearing aids as the latest and greatest since they have the most buttons. They make good gadgets. However, gadget people cannot really be used to support the value of remote control hearing aids. These are the same people who would buy an electric powered turnip if it was a really neat one.

If considering remote control hearing aids, do so on a 30-day trial basis. If they work well and seem worth the cost, only then buy them. If after trying them, the "NO" remote control hearing aid group gains another member, return the hearing aid(s) for a refund and stay with a conventional volume control.

New and Improved

As a society we are conditioned to want the latest and greatest products available. We want the new and concentrated laundry detergent, the newer and faster computer and the car with antilock brakes. Not surprisingly, people with hearing loss want the latest and greatest hearing aids.

The people most interested in cosmetics consider the new completely in the canal (CIC) hearing aids as the greatest. Their greatness is not in more complex or advanced circuitry than is available in larger hearing aids. Their greatness is strictly their small size. A person can wear CIC hearing aids without their being visible to the people around them. It is not that family and friends will be unaware of the hearing aids. Suddenly being able to hear is kind of a dead giveaway. However, barring a bright flashlight and an unusual degree of curiosity, hearing will be the only giveaway.

The programmable hearing aids mentioned earlier also belong in the new and improved category. Aside from the remote control, what makes these hearing aids special is that they can hold multiple memories. In other words, they can be several hearing aids in one. It can be a hearing aid for listening in quiet situations, noisy situations, for listening to music, etc. Just push a button and you are set for that situation. If a person's hearing changes a little bit down the road, the hearing aid fitter can reprogram the aids to compensate for the new hearing levels. It's just another program.

The ultimate in new and improved hearing aids are the new digital ones. These can do everything the programmable aids do and sometimes do more or do it better. Digital hearing aids make use of the same technology that has transformed records into compact disks and is transforming conventional television into digital television. All of this information (sound, picture, whatever) is represented as numbers instead of the old system where information was coded as changes in voltage or current. The output can be modified in an almost infinite number of ways by changing a number here or there. This means a digital hearing aid can be adjusted much like a programmable aid, but more so. They can be used with a wider range of hearing losses, but still be fine tuned very subtly for each user. Digital hearing aids can simply modify sound better than conventional and programmable aids.

It should probably come as no surprise to anyone that since these new and improved hearing aids do more, they also cost more. Sometimes they cost a whole lot more. After the sticker shock, we may be left to wonder whether we really need the new and improved hearing aids. We seemed to do just fine with the old laundry detergent and most of us are still happy with our non-digital televisions. Maybe regular hearing aids might not be so bad after all. Would the new ones really be all that much better? The truth is that many people with mild or simple hearing losses do just fine with conventional hearing aids and don't notice a significant advantage with all this fancy technology. Similarly, a person with long hair that covers their ears may not gain cosmetically by purchasing the smallest hearing aids. In these cases, paying extra for the "latest and greatest" may not always be the best choice.

The point of all this is not that everyone should have completely in the canal, programmable or digital hearing aids. The point is that these new technologies offer great advantages to some people. Those who would have gone without hearing aids for cosmetic reasons, can now wear them. Those who did poorly with hearing aids because they were never quite right for the situations they were in, can now use programmables. Many of the little things about their old hearing aids that drove them nuts (being too loud, not sounding right, etc.) can be overcome or controlled with the new digitals. A person doesn't even have to take the manufacturer's or hearing aid fitter's word that this technology will be a great benefit. They can purchase the hearing aids on a 30-day trial basis and only keep them if they prove to be of benefit.

The Telecoil

In contrast to the completely in the canal, programmable and digital hearing aids that are constantly in newspaper and television advertising, the telecoil is one of the better kept secrets in the hearing aid industry. If forced to describe what a telecoil is or explain its function, most people would have no idea. It could be a top secret device that will make the Star Wars missile defense system possible or it could be a handy dandy tool for snaking telephone wires through walls. How many would know that a telecoil is a little device that can be built into a hearing aid to help a person hear better on the telephone?

Most hearing aid users without a telecoil can attest to the fact that phone usage is a challenge. The primary problem is that whenever a hearing aid is covered up (with a hand, the headset to a telephone, etc.) it will feedback (whistle). This happens when the little bit of sound that normally escapes the ear by leaking around the hearing aid is reflected back into the hearing aid microphone. This reflected sound then becomes amplified again, leaks out of the ear, gets reflected back into the microphone and the process starts over. The hearing aid just keeps amplifying the same sound over and over, getting louder and louder, until all it can do is whistle.

The solution for many is to hold the phone slightly away from the ear so the hearing aid is not directly covered up. This usually solves the feedback problem, but makes it more difficult to hear. Others remove their hearing aid when talking on the phone and do the best they can.

A better solution is the telecoil. This device is built into the hearing aid and picks up the magnetic waves coming off the earpiece of the telephone. It converts the magnetic waves into sound allowing phone usage without making the hearing aid whistle. It also makes the hearing aid compatible with many of the assistive listening devices available in schools, theaters and public buildings. Since the microphone is not being used while the telecoil is on, only the sound from the phone or alternative input device is amplified. Outside noises are blocked out. To use the telecoil, a person simply flips a little switch on their hearing aid and then uses the phone normally. For use with assistive listening devices, a loop of wire is worn around the neck (called a neck loop). This loop is plugged into a sound system, public address system, FM receiver or other input device that generates the magnetic waves picked up by the telecoil.

For a few dollars extra, a telecoil can be built into most new hearing aids at the time of manufacture. It can also be built into older hearing aids, but this is normally a more expensive undertaking. Space is usually the limiting factor in adding a telecoil. If the hearing aid has special or exotic circuitry, there may not be room for a telecoil. Smaller styles such as canal hearing aids usually do not have room for a telecoil. Completely-in-the-canal hearing aids (the really small ones) never have room for a telecoil. However, a telecoil is less likely to be needed since this style is less prone to feedback during telephone use.

As a general rule, if you talk on the phone and a telecoil will fit into your hearing aid, you should have one. A telecoil is a good thing.

Hearing Aid Insurance

Many people buy hearing aids without any thought as to what might later befall these expensive gizmos. Hearing aids come with warranties that protect the user against their quitting or not functioning properly. Extended warranties are available for those who want longer term protection. However, warranties do not usually cover loss or physical damage to the hearing aids. This is where hearing aid insurance takes over. Those who have never lost a set of keys or sat on their sunglasses, might not be interested in hearing aid insurance. For the rest of us, this insurance should be a serious consideration.

Stuff happens! People lose hearing aids. Their small size makes it almost a certainty given enough time. Breakage is another occurrence that can quickly negate a person's hearing aid investment. Hearing aids can break if dropped. Those that do not break may get stepped on or sought out by the vacuum cleaner. People sit on hearing aids, set or drop things on them, close books on them and inadvertently strive in many ways to make them flatter than they were intended to be. Hearing aids also meet their maker having been chewed on, if not actually eaten. People set them next to a bowl of candy or popcorn and wind up accidentally snacking on them. Dogs and cats are also big into chewing up hearing aids. If the hearing aids are not completely shut off before being set down, they may whistle and hurt a dog or cat's ears. Rather than bothering their owner, the pets take care of the problem themselves.

Water is another big hearing aid killer. Hearing aids are electronic devices that are not intended to get wet. Just like it wouldn't be too bright to pour a glass of water into a television set, getting water inside a hearing aid can be unfortunate. The majority of water damage occurs when people forget they are wearing hearing aids. While people like to go swimming and take showers, hearing aids do not. They also do not like riding a shirt or pants pocket into the washing machine. Other water adventures can be experienced by those who choose to change batteries, put in, or take out their hearing aids while sitting on the toilet. This might instead be considered a problem of loss, not damage, should the person inadvertently flush.

All of these things can and do happen to hearing aids. Insuring them against damage or loss is fairly inexpensive and is probably a good investment. Most people that sell hearing aids offer this kind of policy. It may not cover all forms of damage (breakage due to global thermonuclear war, alien invasion, etc.) or all of the incidental expenses involved in replacing a hearing aid, but it should cover most. Another option would be to have the hearing aids included under a home owners or renters insurance policy. This may cover loss (minus any deductible), but not breakage.

Scum Of The Earth

While hearing aids can make the difference between hearing and not hearing, there are a number of negatives generally associated with their purchase and use. The first of these negatives concerns hearing aid fitters. They are generally held in the same high regard as used car salespeople, lawyers and telephone solicitors. In other words, they're seen as the scum of the earth. Like used car salespeople and lawyers, hearing aid fitter services are needed (the need for telephone solicitors is arguable). People just don't want to hear or accept what hearing aid dispensers are telling them and they certainly don't want to pay for it (hearing aids are rarely paid for by insurance). A beginning audiologist once explained to me at length how it was our duty as hearing health care professionals to educate the public and correct this negative stereotype. After considering her words, I told her that life was just too short. It wasn't that I disagreed with her goal, I just considered the chance of achieving it to be pretty remote.

In our society, hearing aids are associated with such things as aging, disability and decline. We don't want to hear that some part of us is broken and can't be fixed. We don't want some kind of device to constantly remind us of this or to point it out to others. We would rather shoot the messenger and walk away.

For those who acknowledge the need for hearing aids, not all accept the limits of what hearing aids can do. Hearing aids can help people to hear better, but they don't restore perfect hearing. Some will focus on the few remaining things they can't hear, rather than enjoy the improvement in what they can hear. Those who do not wear hearing aids may focus on the things a friend that wears hearing aids can't hear, rather than how much better they hear with them. If a person is only willing to consider how they would like things to be, they will never be happy in a world where there are limits. They may consider their hearing aids to be junk because they can't do the impossible.

The vast majority of hearing aid fitters are caring, honest and hard working. Their patients recognize that the hearing aids help them to hear better, but this perception is often outweighed. The fitters are held responsible for the limits of technology, the advertising hype, and for the cost of hearing aids. They also see the hearing aid fitter as a reminder of a hearing disability or handicap that they do not want to accept. Given these perceived negatives, even the best hearing aid fitter is unlikely to be voted man or woman of the year.

Why Do Hearing Aids Cost So Much?

The next big negative associated with hearing aids is their cost. While the price of many consumer electronics is at an all time low, the same cannot be said for hearing aids. Televisions, stereos, microwave ovens, phone answering

134

machines and many other electronic devices cost much less than ten years ago. Video cassette recorders can be purchased for less than half of what they cost when first introduced. Buying a calculator used to be a major expense. Today they are so inexpensive they are displayed next to store check-outs to be purchased as an impulse buy. Although the price of hearing aids may not have increased over the years if inflation is taken into account, it has certainly not dropped in real dollars like other consumer electronics.

What needs to be recognized is that hearing aids are different from other consumer electronics. A company can manufacture a million identical televisions or radios, greatly lowering costs as compared to producing a few at a time. These televisions are then sold by minimum wage employees in discount or department stores. It doesn't work this way with hearing aids. Each hearing aid has to be shaped specifically to fit an individual's ear (for behind-the-ear hearing aids, an earmold has to be specifically shaped to fit the ear). Like dentures, if the fit of a hearing aid is not perfect, pain is often the result. Poor performance and whistling can be other results of an imperfect fit. Further, each hearing aid has to be specifically designed or adjusted to produce an output which compensates for a person's unique hearing loss. A company cannot simply manufacture and sell a million hearing aids in the same way they would televisions. Each hearing aid needs to be made a little bit different from other hearing aids and needs to be prescribed and fitted by trained and experienced people who are not likely to work for minimum wage.

More often than not, the process of fitting a hearing aid costs as much as the hearing aid itself. Initially, there is a hearing test to determine whether a hearing aid is needed and a medical examination to rule out any contraindications to hearing aid use. If a hearing aid is indicated, lengthy counseling is often required to explain hearing aid options, to clarify expectations, and to overcome or at least address the public's generally negative perception of hearing aids and the people who sell them. An impression of the ear is made and sent to the manufacturer along with the specifications for how the aid should sound and what options it should have. Once the manufacturer makes the hearing aid, the fitter checks to make sure it fits the person's ear and works properly. One or more follow-up visits are routinely scheduled to "fine tune" (adjust) the hearing aid(s) to optimize performance and comfort based on the user's experiences with it.

In addition to the manufacturing cost of the hearing aid and the hourly wages of the people involved in fitting it, there are a number of overhead costs that also serve to increase the price to the user. The majority of these costs are the same ones that affect any business: rent, heat, lighting, equipment, etc. The hearing aid practices that can keep these costs lower will need less mark-up on the hearing aids. Hearing aid prices will vary from area to area due to cost of living differences increasing or decreasing overhead costs. Advertising can also drive up the cost. However, if the ads are successful in increasing business, then it can be an advantage for the hearing aid customer. Each hearing aid will not have to cost as much since the price will include a smaller share of the overhead. As a general rule, if you find a hearing aid dispenser that advertises a lot, yet does not appear to have much business, run away. Otherwise, you and a couple other people are likely to pay their bills for that month.

Productivity of the hearing aid fitter can also affect hearing aid costs. If the fitter spends 95% of their time doing "free" hearing tests and telephone soliciting, then the remaining 5% of the time actually spent fitting or repairing hearing aids has to cover all the bills. In contrast, for established practices with good reputations, most of their time is spent maintaining or replacing worn out hearing aids for their previous hearing aid patients. The new people they see are usually referred by their existing hearing aid patients.

Hearing aid customers are not paying them to call up and bother people who do not want hearing aids. Similarly, if part of the hearing aid fitter's overhead is offset by revenue from other audiologic services (diagnostic tests, infant hearing screenings, school hearing screenings, industrial hearing tests, balance testing, etc.), then the mark-up on hearing aids does not have to be as great to cover expenses. If the cost for a particular hearing aid seems out of line with what others you know have paid, or if another fitter quotes a much lower price for the same make and model of hearing aid, then it would be wise to look elsewhere.

One explanation that is sometimes used to explain hearing aid prices is the value or benefit argument. Interestingly, this argument has nothing whatsoever to do with what hearing aids cost. The goal is to convince people that hearing aids are worth what they cost. It goes something like this. Since hearing aids make it easier for hearing impaired children to learn in school, make it possible for adults to remain in the work force, and make it possible for people to maintain active social lives, hearing aids are certainly worth the cost. The alternative is much more expensive in terms of lost learning and earning opportunities, not to mention quality of life issues. This argument sounds good intuitively until we apply it to other goods or services. Few would argue that breakfast is not the most important meal of the day. Children having a good breakfast have been shown to learn more in school, and workers having a good breakfast have been shown to be more productive. If we applied the value theory to breakfast cereal, it would be easy to justify a cost of $10 a bowl. This amount would be a small price to pay for increased productivity. No one would squabble about the $100 a box of cereal would cost, because we would all know that it is worth it. If all our goods and services were priced in this manner, we would be in big trouble. We don't need to start it with hearing aids.

In summary, a lot of reasons are given as to why hearing aids cost so much. Aside from the overhead costs common to any business, there are basically two reasons hearing aids cost more than other retail electronics. The first is that hearing aids have to be custom made both in terms of physical shape and in terms of the electronics used. The second reason is the need for trained and experienced professionals to prescribe an appropriate hearing aid and to fine tune it after the fitting to optimize performance and comfort based on the patient's experiences with it. Unfortunately, rather than accepting these explanations for hearing aid costs, many attribute the high cost to greed on the part of the hearing aid companies and fitters. This of course, takes us back to the scum of the earth viewpoin*.

Batteries Included

Batteries are one of the biggest gripes people have about hearing aids. People gripe about the size, the cost, the freshness, about having to go buy them, having to change them, having to carry spares and how long they last. The color seems OK, but that is about all. Hearing aid batteries do not rate high on most people's list of favorite things. Unlike other battery powered gadgets, hearing aids usually come with the first pack of batteries included. People still do not like them.

All hearing aids use a battery. The battery will generally last one to three weeks, depending on the power of the aid and the circuitry used. Powerful hearing aids will drain batteries much faster than weaker hearing aids. Similarly, if the hearing aid is digitally processing sounds or modifying them some exotic way, the aid will need more power and the battery may not last as long. People are usually horrified that hearing aid batteries do not last the year or more that watch batteries do. However, it must be recognized that all the watch has to do is gradually move its hands around in a circle. The hearing aid has to move the eardrum and ear bones back and forth at hundreds or thousands of times each second. This takes power.

New hearing aid users do not have to go battery shopping for one or two months, since a new hearing aid usually comes with four or more batteries. Additional batteries are available at all of the places where hearing aids are sold and at all kinds of other places that have no apparent connection with hearing aids (drug stores, electronic stores, discount stores, etc.). They usually come in packs of three, four or eight batteries. The average price per battery is about one dollar or slightly more. Some might consider this a lot considering the size of the battery, but it is not an unreasonable amount when compared with what other things cost. People are also concerned about finding the freshest (newest) hearing aid batteries available. However, this concern is often unwarranted because the batteries have a shelf life of several years (provided the little tabs that activate them are not pulled off). Unless the batteries are covered in a foot of dust, they are likely OK.

A few brands of hearing aids incorporate a rechargeable battery as part of their design. These hearing aids are sometimes advertised as not needing conventional batteries. However, they still use a battery, just a different type. The battery needs to be recharged frequently and will eventually wear out and need replaced. Although available for many years, hearing aids that use rechargeable batteries make up only a small part of the hearing aid market. The majority of people opt to use a conventional battery and replace it every couple of weeks, over having to recharge their aid every night and risk going without, should they forget to charge it.

A number of hearing aid fitters have begun to offer free batteries for a year, two years or even for the life of a hearing aid they sell. This does inflate the cost of the hearing aid a little, but eliminates what some people see as a major issue: that they have to buy batteries. The hearing aid fitters that do this have also found that providing free batteries is an effective advertising gimmick.

Feedback

Also on the list of hearing aid negatives is feedback. Feedback is that annoying whistling, screeching or howling that is sometimes heard coming from hearing aids. It can also occur with public address systems, electric guitars and perhaps even with Mr. Microphone if you stand in the wrong place. For the discussion here, however, we are only concerned with hearing aids.

The goal of amplification is to build up a large sound pressure level (loud volume) between the end of the hearing aid and the eardrum. This loud volume moves the eardrum, the ear bones etc. and the person hears. The primary reason that hearing aids feed back, is that the sound which is supposed to go into the ear does not stay there. If it leaks out between the side of the hearing aid and the ear canal wall, it may cause the hearing aid to feed back if the sound goes back into the hearing aid microphone. This escaped sound is again amplified, leaks out of the ear, goes back into the microphone and the process repeats itself over and over until all the hearing aid can do is whistle. Once the feedback starts, it quickly increases to the maximum loudness the hearing aid is capable of producing.

Feedback is most commonly a problem in hearing aids that are very powerful or old. A powerful hearing aid builds up such large sound pressure levels in the ear canal that some of the sound is almost bound to leak out and create feedback. An older hearing aid is more prone to feedback because the ear canal has gradually stretched out around it. This stretching allows space for the sound to leak out. In each of these cases, the solution is to make the hearing aid or hearing aid earmold fit the ear a little better or a little bit tighter.

Another way feedback is likely to occur is when there is a lot of wax in the ear. The sound comes out of the end of the hearing aid and there is nowhere for it to go. The sound hits the earwax and is reflected around the outside of the hearing aid ending up back in the microphone. If the feedback problem is due to earwax, having the wax removed from the ears will solve the problem.

A less common type of feedback is termed internal feedback. This can occur if there is a short in the circuitry causing the feedback or if there is a crack in the hearing aid case which allows the sound to leak directly back to the microphone. Hearing aids with internal feedback whistle, scream and howl just like aids with regular feedback. However, an aid with internal feedback is definitely broken and will likely need to go back to the factory for repair.

Although the sound coming out of a hearing aid is supposed to stay in the ear, there is always at least a little bit that manages to escape. The little bit of sound that does leak out is not a problem unless we cover the ear. Even a normally functioning hearing aid is likely to whistle if we cover the ear. This action reflects the escaping sound back into the microphone. A common example is produce by holding a telephone up to the ear. This is one of the reasons telecoils were invented.

Some of the newer and more exotic hearing aids are designed to recognize when they are starting to feed back and to stop the process before it really gets going. Unfortunately, this may sometimes mean that the hearing aid reduces the overall volume. The feedback will be gone, but the person may not hear optimally due to the volume on the aid not being loud enough.

While feedback is a nuisance, it can usually be controlled or eliminated provided the aid is the appropriate style and is fit properly. Some styles of hearing aids will be less prone to feedback than others. Larger or longer hearing aids and earmolds may have fewer feedback problems because it is

141

harder for the sound to leak out around them. Behind-the-ear hearing aids are less prone to feedback because the microphone is further from the ear canal. Feedback is not likely to be much of a problem for people with mild hearing losses regardless of hearing aid style because there is less sound pressure to leak out of the ear. Style becomes a more important consideration with more severe hearing losses. The physical fit of the hearing aid or earmold is very important because if it is off even a little bit the sound will leak out and cause feedback. Hearing aid fitters can usually avoid, or when they do occur, solve feedback problems by selecting an appropriate aid in the first place or by adjusting the fit if it is off a little.

These issues of selecting the appropriate hearing aids and making them fit properly to reduce or eliminate the likelihood of feedback, illustrate why it is so important to find an experienced hearing aid fitter and let them do things properly. Let them tell you what style of aid will work for your hearing loss and then follow their recommendations. If the hearing aids do feed back, return to the fitter to see if the feedback can be reduced or eliminated. Most of the time it can.

Bags, Boxes and Drawers Of Hearing Aids

The final common objection to amplification is having known someone who has had bags, boxes and drawers of hearing aids, and they don't wear any of them. The majority of people with hearing aids wear them and do their best to make them live long enough to extract their money's worth. Others buy hearing aids just to have them sit in a box or dresser drawer. They do not start out with the goal of buying hearing aids for their furniture, but it can work out this way. The two biggest reasons for this are not having wanted them in the first place or not being completely satisfied with how their hearing aids work.

Some people buy hearing aids only because it is what their friends or family want them to do. They may not want hearing aids or feel they need them, but still buy them anyway. Given this level of motivation, it is not too surprising that they might not wear them. When their friends or family are around or when they are nagged about it, they may wear their hearing aids a little, but otherwise, the hearing aids live in a drawer.

Other people buy, but do not wear their hearing aids, because they do not like something about them. They might sound too soft, loud, tinny, rumbly or whistle while in the ears. The fit of the hearing aids might be off, making them uncomfortable or causing them to fall out of the ears. Even if the hearing aids make it possible to hear better, a person is not likely to wear them if they are considered more nuisance than help.

Hearing aids are usually sold with a 30-day trial period and a one or two year warranty. If, at the end of the trial period the person does not think they are going to wear the hearing aids, they should not keep them. If the hearing aids help, but there is something annoying or disappointing about them, they should talk with the hearing aid fitter to see if it can be corrected or at least improved. Unfortunately, many people keep hearing aids they do not intend to wear. They might be shy about returning them or may not have realized that they had, or should have had, a 30-day trial. Experienced hearing aid fitters understand that a certain number of people will return their hearing aids (even when they work well and are as good as possible for that person's hearing loss). People may also be shy about pointing out to the hearing aid fitter any problems they are having. It is not unusual for a set of hearing aids to need some fine tuning after being initially fit. If the wearer does not go back to point out any problem(s), there is no chance that they will get better.

Worse than the people who keep but do not wear their hearing aids and the people who should, but did not, have their hearing aids adjusted, are the ones who just keep buying more and more hearing aids. These are the people with bags, boxes and drawers of hearing aids. They do not return trial hearing aids they will not wear or have their unsatisfactory hearing aids adjusted. They just keep buying new hearing aids. Quite often, they get the latest ones (this also means the most expensive) with the expectation that they will be vastly better from the ones before. We have had patients complain about their past experiences and then show us $10,000 or more worth of hearing aids lovingly enclosed in a paper sack. Surprisingly, rather than this having scared them off, many of these people want to buy still more hearing aids.

To avoid bags, boxes and drawers of hearing aids, a person should not keep hearing aids they do not intend to wear. They should also not replace hearing aids that work just fine, simply because someone says they are old or that new ones might work better. If a person is not satisfied with an older set of hearing aids and a hearing aid fitter says they can do better, the fitter should be held accountable if the new ones do not work better. Try the new aids, but do not keep them unless they are clearly better that the ones being replaced. If the old ones work as well, why spend money on new?

Beyond Hearing Aids: The Cochlear Implant

Some hearing losses can be so severe that not even hearing aids will help. Only a few years ago these people would have been totally out of luck. Today it is possible to return many of them to a world of sound through the use of a cochlear implant.

A cochlear implant is a device that provides or restores hearing to severely or profoundly hearing impaired individuals by electrically stimulating the few remaining nerve cells in the inner ear. Part of the device is surgically implanted and part is worn externally. The external part is about the size of a pack of cigarettes (some of the newest ones are much smaller) and is powered by one or two batteries. It picks up surrounding sounds through a small microphone, codes and transforms the sound into magnetic waves and transmits them across the skin to the internal device. The internal device picks up the magnetic waves, transforms them into electricity and delivers it to the inner ear through several small electrodes (wires). The magnetic waves also serve to power the internal device so that it does not require a batterry. The body of the inner part is smaller than a pack of matches and is implanted within the bone behind the ear. The implant detects surrounding sounds, converts them into electric signals and supplies these signals to the inner ear. All that is left is for the remaining nerve pathways to transmit these signals to the brain so the person can hear.

A cochlear implant does not restore normal hearing. It would be unreasonable to expect an implant's limited number of electrodes (usually about 22 at the time of this writing) to work as well as the thousands of nerve cells in a healthy ear. An implant can restore the awareness of sound, the loudness, pattern and pitch of sound, and in many cases, speech understanding (even without lip-reading). The hearing with a cochlear implant may not be perfect, but it is a whole lot better than not hearing.

While it can restore hearing to many, a cochlear implant is not for everyone. People with mild or moderate hearing losses are better served with hearing aids. Only if a hearing loss is deemed severe or profound would an implant be considered and only then if hearing aids had already been tried and were not helpful. The worst candidates for a cochlear implant are adults who never learned speech and language and have no memory of sound. An implant could still provide sound to these people, but it would be largely meaningless beyond simple sound awareness or pattern perception. These people would already have developed some other mode of communication (sign language, gestures, etc.)

and since they are beyond the childhood years where it is easiest to learn speech and language, the odds of an implant helping them to develop or make effective use of speech and language is very low.

The best candidates for an implant are people who once heard well but lost their hearing. They already have an understanding of language and what speech should sound like. Even if the implant does not provide them with a perfect or complete reproduction of what a person may say, their experience and knowledge of language often lets them fill in the gaps. Young children with severe or profound hearing losses are also considered good cochlear implant candidates. By using the implant to provide sound during the language formative years, many of these children can develop normal or near-normal speech and language skills (provided extensive speech and language therapy). Without the implant, this would be unlikely.

A cochlear implant is not for the faint of wallet. Once the cost of the evaluation, the device, the surgery, the follow-up programming and maintenance are taken into account, a person could buy a really nice luxury car for what one of these things costs.

Cochlear implants have become recognized as useful and are considered very cost effective when compared against other medical devices. Although new ones are always being developed, cochlear implants in general, are no longer considered experimental devices. This means that medical insurance may now cover part or all of the cost. Some severely or profoundly hearing impaired people who do not have insurance or have insurance that does not cover cochlear implants still decide to proceed with an implant and pay for it themselves. For them, the cost of not hearing is what is unjustifiable.

Conclusion

A Hearing Bias

By now it should be pretty clear a definite bias exists throughout this book that hearing is better than not hearing. We have not been overly subtle in our statements that when possible, hearing losses should be corrected: especially bad ones.

People with hearing loss live in a smaller world than they might think. Physically their world is the same as other people's, but with reduced hearing, there is less of it they are aware of, or able to interact with. If they can't hear the phone ringing, they won't know there is a person at the other end. If they can't hear the doorbell, they won't see who is there. If they can't hear well enough to understand people on the television or on the phone, then benefit from all of the people and information available here is lost. A severe enough hearing loss can reduce a person's world to only those individuals who stand directly in front of them and shout. It could be argued that their vision would keep their world large by helping to compensate for the hearing loss. However, the speaker would have to be in view, the person would have to be aware that someone was talking and they would have to be able to lip-read well. It could happen, but, normally it does not.

Many of the hearing impaired who have their hearing improved through surgery or hearing aids are surprised to find out how small their world had become. They rediscover that the refrigerator makes noise, the microwave beeps when done, the toilet makes noise when flushed, that cars are not really quiet inside and that it was their hearing loss that kept them from hearing the birds outside. They are aware of the phone when it rings and can tell the solicitor at the other end that they do not want to change phone companies, get a magazine subscription, have the basement waterproofed or invest in a commemorative limited edition Elvis toilet seat. All of a sudden their world is populated by people who do not mumble and who can be understood. They can understand people who are talking to them as well as people who are talking to others. If someone calls from another room, they will be aware of it and can go have a conversation or not depending on their mood. Their world now includes more than the one person shouting in their face.

We understand and respect that some people may choose not to hear. However, the people we see in our practice and most likely those of you reading this book are motivated to hear. You want to set your own limits, not have a hearing loss do it for you. Consequently, our bias in favor of hearing should not be too much of a problem. For anyone who might be concerned about our bias, rest assured that we do not generally drag people in off the street and force them to hear.

Motivation And Expectation

Although a person's expectations and level of motivation may have little or nothing to do with their hearing loss, they do have a great impact on what can or should be done about it. A person who does not think that they have a hearing loss or are not motivated to find out, are unlikely to have their ears checked in the first place. Similarly, if they suspect a hearing problem but do not think anything can be done to correct it, they are also unlikely to seek help. If a relative, friend or coworker manages to drag one of these people to an ear specialist, this person is likely to be less than enthusiastic about the evaluation. If diagnosed with a hearing loss, they may choose to disregard the findings or not follow the recommendations.

The effect of a person's motivation can often be seen in their success or failure with hearing aid use. If a person does not feel they have a hearing problem, they are not going to be motivated to wear hearing aids. No matter how good the hearing aids may be or how much they can improve the person's hearing, they are useless if not worn. A person has to want to hear better.

People who have incorrect or unrealistic expectations about hearing aids may be less likely to try them or to do well with the ones they have. Further, even if the hearing aids do help, they may be unhappy if their expectation is that the aids will restore perfect hearing. Others will be unhappy if hearing aids do not filter out every unwanted noise, improve everyone's diction or guarantee they'll always be able to hear a pin drop. Hearing professionals counsel people about realistic expectations and try to educate them about what is and is not possible. Some of these people are very willing to modify their views in light of new information, others are not. The latter make very unhappy hearing aid users (or non-users) because they want the impossible and are not willing to recognize it as such.

The effect of motivation and expectations on hearing impaired people are not just limited to hearing aid use. A motivated person is more likely to pursue a surgery that could improve their hearing. A motivated person is more likely to schedule follow-up appointments to control chronic conditions (ear infections, earwax, etc.) that might affect the hearing. They are also more likely to develop and use listening strategies to improve their hearing or understanding in the situations where they have problems. As with hearing aids, people in these situations having unrealistic expectations are less likely to follow through with what they started or to be satisfied with the results.

Ear professionals try to understand how much a person wants to hear better (motivation) and how well they understand what is possible (expectations), because these must be taken into account when deciding on an appropriate treatment. There is little point in selling hearing aids to a person with a mild hearing loss if they feel their hearing is fine. They won't wear them. An ear surgery that needs to be followed by several weeks of special care or limited physical activity would be inappropriate for someone unwilling to comply with the limitations.

When a person lacks motivation or has unrealistic expectations, the best course of action can often be to wait. If, at some later time they decide they want to hear better and are willing to understand what can and cannot be done, then interventions (surgery, medication, hearing aids, listening strategies etc.) are more likely to be judged as successful. Until then, it is not possible for either the individual or doctor to win.

Final Thoughts

This is the part of the book where everyone is expecting or hoping for some universal "truth" or great insight about hearing loss. After seeing thousands of patients with varying degrees of hearing loss, we have found they do share a similar "truth" about having a hearing loss. They would rather not have one. In fact, they are often extremely clear in expressing that they do not consider hearing loss a good thing.

The reason hearing loss is not a good thing is that it can make more difficult, or severely limit, what a person does. It is hard to watch a movie when you can't understand the dialog. Enjoying the company of family and friends is more difficult when conversations are misheard or seem unclear. Students have a harder time in school if they can't understand what the teacher is saying. The workplace becomes a tougher place in which to function effectively, and in some cases, a more dangerous place to work. A hearing loss may not prevent people from living happy, healthy and productive lives. But, in a hearing world, the loss can make it much more difficult.

Complicating the listening difficulties caused by a hearing loss is the fact that most people are not well prepared to deal with it. We tend to be so ignorant of the entire subject that we have no idea who to ask for help or how much to believe the information or recommendations we may receive.

Also complicating the difficulties caused by a hearing loss are the generally negative implications or stereotypes (aging, disability, etc.) associated with this impairment. Because of this, people try to ignore or deny a hearing loss as long as possible. They do not want to accept or have anyone else know that they have a hearing loss for fear these negative stereotypes might be applied to them. Rather than being seen as a disease, as a natural process or simply as bad luck, many people act as if hearing loss is something to hide or be ashamed of. As a result, many will insist on the smallest hearing aids on the market, even if they are not the most appropriate for their hearing loss. They are more concerned with not looking hearing impaired than not being hearing impaired.

The "truth" we would like the reader to take away from this book is that hearing loss is not something to hide or be ashamed of. It is something to correct when possible, or compensate for when not medically correctable. Modern medical and surgical techniques have made it possible to improve or restore hearing for many who would have remained hearing impaired or deaf years ago. Hearing aids and assistive listening technology are constantly evolving, making it possible for more people with hearing loss to hear well and to hear comfortably. We agree with our patients that hearing loss is not a good thing. However, their realization is only of value if it motivates them to do something about the hearing loss. We hope you have found this book informative and useful toward this end.

Glossary

Acoustic Reflex - A reflex in the middle ear that produces a stiffening of the eardrum in response to loud sounds.

Adventitious Hearing Loss - A hearing loss occurring sometime after birth.

Air-Bone Gap - Any difference between how a person should hear and how they actually hear if some of the sound is being lost as it passes through the middle ear.

Analog Hearing Aids - A hearing aid that processes sound as a voltage. All of the older hearing aids work this way.

Assistive Listening Device - Any device that makes it easier for a person to hear or be aware of sound.

Audiogram - A graph of a person's hearing levels.

Audiologist - A person university trained in the performance and interpretation of ear and hearing related tests. Audiologists also prescribe, fit and evaluate hearing aids and assistive listening devices.

Audiology - The study or science of hearing.

Audiometry - The performance of hearing related tests.

Auditory Brainstem Response (ABR) Testing - A test that measures the brain's response to a series of clicking sounds. The test can be used to calculate hearing or rule out problems along the hearing nerve.

Auditory Processing Disorder - A hearing problem in which some of the understanding or clarity (not volume) of sound is lost within the brain or nerve pathways leading to the brain.

Aural Rehabilitation - Training to help individuals compensate for a hearing loss.

Automatic Gain Control (AGC) - A form of hearing aid circuitry that monitors the volume of sound so it remains within a comfortable range for the hearing aid wearer.

Background Noise - Any sound that a person does not wish to hear or that interferes with what they are trying to hear.

Behavioral Observation Audiometry (BOA) - A hearing test used with infants. Their behavior is observed to see how they respond to sound.

Behind The Ear (BTE) Hearing Aid - The body of this form of hearing aid hangs behind the ear. Sound from the aid is carried through a small clear tube to an earmold that fits snugly into the ear.

Binaural - Both ears.

Body Aid - The largest and most powerful of the conventional hearing aids. The body of this form of hearing aid is about the size of a pack of cigarettes and can be worn on the belt or in a pocket. Sound is carried from the aid through a small wire that leads to an earpiece.

Bone Conduction - Hearing produced by sound vibrating the skull in relation to the hearing nerves, rather than the nerves moving while the skull remains still. This is largely how we hear our own voice.

Bone Conduction Hearing Aid - A hearing aid that vibrates the skull to produce hearing.

Canal Hearing Aid - A hearing aid that fits entirely within the ear canal.

Cerumen - Earwax.

Cholesteatoma - A disease where skin cells grow uncontrolled through a hole in the eardrum and accumulate in the middle ear. This often causes infection and damage to the surrounding structures.

Closed Captioning - Printed text at the bottom of movies or television detailing the events and dialog occurring on screen.

Cochlea - The organ of hearing.

Cochlear Implant - An electronic device that is surgically implanted into the inner ear to restore sound to severely and profoundly hearing impaired individuals.

Completely In The Canal (CIC) Hearing Aid - The smallest of the in the canal hearing aids.

Compression - A form of automatic gain control in a hearing aid that keeps sounds from becoming uncomfortably loud.

Conditioned Audiometry - A type of hearing testing used with young children. Children are operantly or classically conditioned to perform some activity (dropping a block in a box, pressing a toy button, etc.) in response to sounds.

Conductive Hearing Loss - A form of hearing loss caused by the outer or middle ear blocking or not effectively transmitting sound to the inner ear.

Congenital Hearing Loss - A hearing loss present from birth.

CROS (Contralateral Routing Of Signal) Hearing Aid – A hearing aid designed for a person who has hearing in only one ear. The aid picks up sound on the non-hearing side and transmits it to the better ear.

Decibels (dB) - The loudness units hearing level and hearing loss are measured in.

Digital Hearing Aids - Hearing aids that process sounds as numbers instead of as a voltage. This is the way CD players and digital television work.

Disarticulation - A break or separation in the middle ear bones.

Discrimination - Hearing clarity or the ability to understand speech.

Dynamic Range - The range of loudness between the softest sounds that a person can hear and the sounds that are uncomfortably loud.

Eardrum Perforation - A hole in the eardrum.

Ear Impression - An impression or cast of the ear canal used to make a hearing aid or earplugs.

Earmold - The portion of a behind the ear hearing aid that fits into the ear.

ENT - Ear Nose and Throat doctor.

Etiology - The cause of a problem, disease, pathology, etc...

Eustachian Tube - A small passageway leading from the back of the throat to the middle ear that supplies air and equalizes pressure in the middle ear.

Feedback - The whistling that occurs when the sound coming out of a hearing aid leaks out of the ear, goes back into the hearing aid microphone and gets amplified over and over.

FM System - An assistive listening device that picks up a speaker's voice through a microphone and transmits it, using radio waves, to a person wearing a special receiver unit. The device effectively moves the listener's ears right up to the mouth of the person speaking.

Frequency - The pitch of a sound.

Hearing Aid Trial - A period of time (usually 30 days) during which a person may try hearing aids that were custom made for them. If unsatisfied for any reason, the person should be able to return them for a refund (minus an agreed upon trial fee).

Hertz - The frequency or pitch of a sound.

Idiopathic - Having an unknown cause.

Incus - The center most of the three middle ear bones.

ITE Hearing Aid - The general abbreviation for any In-The-Ear hearing aid.

Linear Hearing Aids - These amplify sound by a set amount (i.e. 20%, 30%, etc.)   at any particular pitch; regardless of the initial volume. This can result in a sound that was already very loud becoming amplified even more.

Lip-Reading - Watching the mouth of a person speaking as a method to help understand their words.

Listening Strategy - Any method or plan that helps a person to hear in a particular situation.

Malleus - The outermost of the three middle ear bones.

Masking - Any sound that serves to cover up another.

Meniere's Disease - A syndrome characterized by vertigo, tinnitus, fullness in the ear and a fluctuating hearing loss.

Mild Hearing Loss - A 20% to 40% hearing loss.

Moderate Hearing Loss - A 40% to 60% hearing loss.

Monaural - One ear.

Most Comfortable Loudness Level (MCL) - The volume at which sounds are most comfortable.

Myringotomy - A small incision made in the eardrum by a physician to drain infection or fluid from the middle ear.

Nerve Damage - Damage to the hair (nerve) cells in the Inner ear.

Non-Linear Hearing Aids - Hearing aids that amplify soft sounds by a different amount than loud sounds in order to keep the volume comfortable to the wearer.

Ossicles - General term referring to the three middle ear bones.

Ossiculoplasty - Surgery to repair or replace one or more of the middle ear bones.

Otalgia - Ear pain.

Otitis Media - Fluid or infection in the middle ear.

Otolaryngology - The medical specialty that deals with problems of the ear, nose, throat, head and neck.

Otology - The medical specialty that deals with ear and hearing problems.

Otorrhea - Drainage from the ear.

Otosclerosis - An ear disease that produces areas of spongy bone that can fix the smallest of the middle ear bones (the stapes) in place. This results in a conductive hearing loss.

Otoscope - A specialized flashlight for examining the ear.

Ototoxic - Any substance or medication that may damage hearing.

Permanent Threshold Shift (PTS) - A permanent worsening in hearing due to noise exposure.

Post-lingual - After language development.

Pre-lingual - Before language development.

Presbycusis - A group of ear related problems that can cause hearing loss as we age.

Pressure Equalization (PE) Tube - A small tube that is surgically inserted in the eardrum to allow air into the middle ear when the eustachian tube is not functioning.

Profound Hearing Loss - Essentially a total hearing loss.

Pure Tone Testing - This test measures the softest level a person can hear at a number of different pitches.

Recruitment - The phenomenon whereby loud sounds can seem as loud for a hearing impaired person as for a person with normal hearing.

Selective Amplification - The general method used for fitting hearing aids in which more power is provided at the pitches where a person has greater hearing loss and less power is provided at the pitches where the hearing is closer to normal.

Sensorineural Hearing Loss - A hearing loss caused by damage to the hair (nerve) cells in the inner ear.

Severe Hearing Loss - An 80% to 100% hearing loss.

Sign Language - A method of communication in which hand and body gestures are used rather than spoken words.

Speech Reception Threshold (SRT) - The quietest level at which a person can understand simple two syllable words.

Stapes - The smallest of the middle ear bones.

Stapedectomy - A surgical procedure that removes all or part of a stapes bone that has been fixed in place by otosclerosis and replaces it with a prosthesis.

Telecoil - A device built into many hearing aids that make it easier to hear on the phone.

Temporary Threshold Shift (TTS) - A temporary (lasting less than a day) hearing loss due to exposure to loud sounds. Repeated exposure to sounds loud enough to cause TTS can eventually lead to permanent hearing loss.

Tinnitus - A perceived ringing, roaring or cricket-like sound in the ear.

Tympanic Membrane - The eardrum.

Tympanogram - A graph that shows whether the eardrum is intact and how well it moves.

Tympanoplasty - Surgery to repair or replace a damaged eardrum.

Uncomfortable Loudness Level (UCL) - The volume at which sounds become uncomfortably loud.

Vent - A small hole through a hearing aid or earmold that lets air into the ear.

Acknowledgments

We wish to thank all of the members of the Warren Otologic Group. Although not every member may have contributed directly to this book, over the years, each has contributed to the ideas and philosophy of patient care that are expressed here. We also have to recognize all of those who taught us or gave us the opportunity to build on their knowledge and experience.

About The Authors

John M. Burkey, M.A. is a clinical audiologist who evaluates and counsels people with hearing loss or suspected hearing loss. He is certified by the American Speech Language and Hearing Association and is a Fellow of the American Academy of Audiology. He is licensed to practice audiology in Ohio and Pennsylvania. He has authored, co-authored or contributed to articles for hearing, hearing aid and medical journals.

William H. Lippy, M.D., Arnold G. Schuring, M.D. and Franklin M. Rizer, M.D. are otologists who diagnose and treat ear and hearing problems. All three physicians are certified by the American Board of Otolaryngology and are Fellows of the American Academy of Otolaryngology - Head and Neck Surgery. Each physician has published and lectured extensively on ear and hearing related subjects.

All of the authors are members of the Warren Otologic Group; a medical practice founded by William H. Lippy, M.D. in 1960. It is comprised of physicians, nurses, audiologists, speech pathologists, technicians and support staff all dedicated to the diagnosis and treatment of hearing loss, ear diseases, balance disorders and problems of the head and neck. It is one of the leading centers in the world for cochlear implants to treat nerve deafness and for stapedectomy surgery to improve or correct hearing losses due to otosclerosis. The practice is highly dedicated to research into the effectiveness of current medical and surgical techniques as well as developing new treatments for ear disease and hearing loss.